MCQs and OSCEs for the Primary FRCA

BARTS AND THE LONDON
SCHOOL OF MEDICINE AND DENTISTRY
WHITECHAPEL LIBRARY,TURNER STREET, LONDON E1 2AD
020 7882 7110

ONE WEEK LOAN
Book are to be returned on or before the last date below,
otherwise fines may be charged.

MCQs and OSCEs for the Primary FRCA

Edward Doyle FRCA

Consultant Anaesthetist,
Royal Hospital for Sick Children, Edinburgh, UK.

Paul Goggin MB BS FANZCA

Consultant Anaesthetist,
Royal Infirmary of Edinburgh, UK.

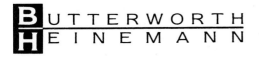

BUTTERWORTH
HEINEMANN

Butterworth-Heinemann
Linacre House, Jordan Hill, Oxford OX2 8DP
A division of Reed Educational and Professional Publishing Ltd

A member of the Reed Elsevier plc group

OXFORD   BOSTON   JOHANNESBURG
MELBOURNE   NEW DELHI   SINGAPORE

First published 1997

British Library Cataloguing in Publication Data
A catalogue record for this book is available from the British Library

ISBN 0 7506 2338 1

Composition by Genesis Typesetting, Laser Quay, Rochester, Kent
Printed and bound by Hartnolls Ltd, Bodmin, Cornwall

Contents

Introduction   vii

How to sit a multiple choice question examination   ix

EXAM NO. 1
Questions   1
Answers   15

EXAM NO. 2
Questions   30
Answers   44

EXAM NO. 3
Questions   58
Answers   72

EXAM NO. 4
Questions   86
Answers   100

EXAM NO. 5
Questions   114
Answers   130

OSCEs
Questions   144
Answers   148

Index   151

Introduction

The multiple choice component of the recently introduced College of Anaesthetists Primary examination is made up of 90 MCQs to be completed in 3 hours. Having successfully passed this step, candidates are then invited to take OSCE (Objective Structured Clinical Examination) questions and two 30-minute vivas. The multiple choice paper is the obvious initial goal and will offer a considerable hurdle for those unfamiliar or lacking in confidence with the format.

The aim of this book is *not* to pre-empt the questions which will appear in the examination. The questions in this book have been designed to cover a wide range of topics, to impart important information about topics and to act as a prompt for further reading. The 'Answers' sections give brief explanations and, where appropriate, references for the topic.

As such, these MCQs should be used as part of a study plan. Candidates should attempt them as soon as they begin preparing for the examination and not wait until they feel they have enough information to tackle them. This book can then act as a means of identifying gaps in the candidate's knowledge on major topics.

There are five papers in this book made up of 60 questions each. The topic mix reflects that of the actual MCQ paper, namely pharmacology, physiology, biochemistry, clinical anaesthesia, physics, clinical measurement, and statistics. Following the MCQs, is a set of OSCEs to attempt. These will act as a further guide to the type of study required.

How to sit a multiple choice question examination

MCQs can be a cause of considerable anxiety for many candidates while others see them as 'easy pickings'. Although it might be true that in a multiple choice question, 'the answer is right there in front of you', it is essential to read the questions *very* carefully before committing oneself to an answer. In no other written examination is the time required actually to write the answer so short, so most of the 3 hours is to be spent reading the questions. Do so carefully and deliberately, but don't dwell on questions for too long if they are not obvious. However, if you do skip questions on your initial run-through of the paper, be very careful not to get out of sequence on the answer sheet.

Don't become hung-up on the wording of questions. The examiners spend much time on removing any ambiguity in the construction of questions. If, despite the best attempts to vet such questions, there is one that is obviously flawed, it will usually be removed from the pool of questions after the examination and not counted toward your total. Be careful with the timing of questions and don't dwell or panic when you are stuck. Even as the best candidate, you are highly unlikely to answer all the questions correctly, so move on and make the most of the ones you can answer. Once again, be very careful when you do temporarily pass over questions that you don't get out of sequence on the answer sheet. Good luck.

Exam no. 1   Questions

1. **Concerning humidity:**
   a) The factor which determines the amount of water vapour which a given volume of air can contain is the temperature.
   b) As the temperature rises, the amount of water vapour which a given volume of air can contain falls.
   c) The absolute humidity is the maximum amount of water vapour which a given volume of air can hold at a given temperature.
   d) Relative humidity is the ratio of the mass of water vapour present in a given volume of air to the mass of water vapour required to saturate the same volume of air at the same temperature.
   e) Relative humidity may be expressed as the ratio of actual vapour pressure of water present to the saturated vapour pressure which is obtained at the same temperature.

2. **When a fluid flows through a tube of varying diameter:**
   a) Flow is a manifestation of kinetic energy.
   b) Pressure is a manifestation of potential energy.
   c) At the constriction of a Venturi device, flow increases.
   d) At the constriction of a Venturi device, pressure increases.
   e) The Venturi principle applies only to gases.

3. **An inaccurate SpO_2 reading may be given by a pulse oximeter in the presence of:**
   a) Carboxyhaemoglobin.
   b) Methaemoglobin.
   c) Fetal haemoglobin (HbF).
   d) Bilirubin.
   e) Methylene blue.

4. The performance of the following oxygen delivery devices is dependent on the patient's respiratory pattern:
a) Nasal cannulae.
b) Hudson mask.
c) Ventimask.
d) Bain anaesthetic circuit.
e) Headbox.

5. In a recording of a 12-lead ECG:
a) Twelve electrodes are used.
b) Leads I, II and III are unipolar leads.
c) Lead II usually gives a particularly good trace of atrial electrical activity because it is parallel to the direction of atrial depolarization.
d) Electrical activity of the heart in an antero-posterior direction is detected by the praecordial leads.
e) The bipolar leads measure the voltage difference between two electrodes while unipolar leads measure the voltage at an electrode relative to a reference taken as zero.

6. Human neurotransmitters include:
a) Glycine.
b) Adrenaline.
c) Substance P.
d) Acetylcholine.
e) Vitamin A.

7. Prolactin:
a) Is secreted from the hypothalamus.
b) Is a glycoprotein in structure.
c) Prevents ovulation in lactating women.
d) Secretion is stimulated by dopamine.
e) Inhibits lactation.

8. Luteinizing hormone:
a) Is a glycoprotein dimer secreted by the posterior pituitary.
b) Increases testosterone secretion.
c) Is required for full maturation of ovarian follicles.
d) Is the final stimulation to ovulation.
e) Acts via intracellular cyclic AMP.

9. **The following reduce the glomerular filtration rate:**
   a) Mean arterial blood pressure of <120 mmHg.
   b) Ureteric obstruction.
   c) Glomerulonephritis.
   d) Mannitol.
   e) Angiotensin II.

10. **In the renal tubules there is absorption of:**
   a) Sodium.
   b) Urea.
   c) Glucose.
   d) Bicarbonate.
   e) Inulin.

11. **The oxygen–haemoglobin dissociation curve:**
   a) In healthy adults has a P_{50} value of 3.4 kPa.
   b) Is moved to the left by a fall in pH.
   c) Is moved to the right by a fall in temperature.
   d) In the fetus has a lower P_{50} than in the adult.
   e) Is moved to the right by an increase in the 2,3-diphosphoglycerate (2,3-DPG) concentration in erythrocytes.

12. **Magnesium:**
   a) Has a normal plasma concentration of 3–5 mmol/l.
   b) 99% in the body is intracellular.
   c) When deficient may cause muscle weakness and dysrhythmias.
   d) Potentiates the action of Ca^{2+} at the neuromuscular junction.
   e) When supplementation is required must be given intravenously, since it is not absorbed enterally.

13. **The following coagulation factors are common to the intrinsic and extrinsic pathways:**
   a) Thrombin.
   b) Factor X.
   c) Factor VIII.
   d) Thromboplastin.
   e) Protein C.

14. Renal blood flow:
   a) Is assessed by inulin clearance.
   b) In health is about 20% of cardiac output.
   c) Is directed mainly to the renal medulla.
   d) Is pressure dependent.
   e) Is increased by NSAIDs.

15. The following factors contribute to the alveolar to arterial pO_2 gradient:
   a) Right to left shunt.
   b) Ventilation/perfusion mismatch.
   c) Respiratory quotient.
   d) Cardiac output.
   e) Haemoglobin concentration.

16. The following types of compounds act as neurotransmitters:
   a) Amines.
   b) Steroids.
   c) Peptides.
   d) Amino acids.
   e) Acetylcholine.

17. Neutrophils:
   a) Contain cytoplasmic granules which contain inflammatory mediators.
   b) Have a mean half-life in the circulation of 24 h.
   c) Absorb many bacteria by the process of phagocytosis.
   d) Produce the oxygen radicals O_2^- and H_2O_2 as bactericidal agents.
   e) Develop into tissue macrophages.

18. The aminoglycoside antibiotics:
   a) Are active against Gram positive organisms.
   b) Are absorbed from the gut.
   c) Should not be used in patients with renal failure.
   d) May impair neuromuscular transmission by competing with acetylcholine at its receptors.
   e) Inhibit the synthesis of bacterial DNA.

19. Compared with fentanyl, alfentanil:
a) Has a smaller volume of distribution and a longer terminal elimination half-life.
b) Has a quicker onset of action.
c) Is less lipid soluble.
d) Has a lower pK_a.
e) Is less potent.

20. Adenosine:
a) Is a coronary vasoconstrictor.
b) Has a negative inotropic effect.
c) Has a half-life in plasma of 5–10 min.
d) Is metabolized in the liver.
e) Is primarily used for the termination of supraventricular tachycardias.

21. Heparin:
a) Inhibits the action of antithrombin III.
b) Is monitored using the prothrombin time.
c) Is contraindicated during pregnancy.
d) Has a half-life in the plasma of 30–60 min.
e) May be reversed using protamine sulphate.

22. The following drugs are phospodiesterase inhibitors:
a) Dopexamine.
b) Enoximone.
c) Sodium nitroprusside.
d) Milrinone.
e) Aminophylline.

23. The following drug interactions are pharmacodynamic in nature:
a) Penicillin and gentamicin against *Streptococcus viridans*.
b) Verapamil and atenolol.
c) Gentamicin and non-depolarizing muscle relaxants.
d) Alcohol and warfarin.
e) Diuretics and lithium.

24. Aspirin (acetylsalicylic acid) is indicated for:
   a) Primary prevention of cardiac and cerebral vascular occlusion.
   b) As an antipyretic in children.
   c) Treatment of deep venous thrombosis.
   d) Secondary prevention of myocardial infarction.
   e) Arthritis.

25. Morphine sulphate:
   a) Produces a reduction in central neural activity.
   b) Acts mostly via presynaptic inhibition of neurotransmitter release.
   c) Increases potassium conductance across neuronal membranes and causes hyperpolarization.
   d) Has effects in the peripheral nervous system.
   e) Exerts its actions via G-protein coupled receptors.

26. Benzodiazepines:
   a) Are extensively excreted in the urine.
   b) Are highly protein bound.
   c) When used chronically, induce hepatic microsomal enzymes.
   d) Are antalgesic.
   e) Cross the placenta.

27. Volatile anaesthetics:
   a) Increase in potency when fluorine replaces chlorine on hydrocarbon molecules.
   b) Tend to increase in potency as molecular weight increases within a series of similar molecules.
   c) Increase in potency when bromine replaces chlorine.
   d) Have an MAC which tends to increase with age.
   e) Tend to be more soluble in blood when fluorine is the halogen present in the compound rather than bromine or chlorine.

28. In a healthy 3 year old child undergoing nephrectomy, the following are true:
   a) The weight is about 16 kg.
   b) The circulating blood volume is about 3000 ml.
   c) An appropriate induction dose of thiopentone is 75–100 mg.
   d) A cuffed 5.0 mm endotracheal tube should be tried initially.
   e) Epidural analgesia is contraindicated.

29. The following have been shown to reduce the incidence of deep venous thrombosis after surgery:
   a) Warfarin.
   b) Aspirin.
   c) Intravenous infusion of heparin.
   d) Intraoperative infusion of 7–15 ml/kg dextran 70.
   e) Diclofenac sodium.

30. Epiglottitis:
   a) May be caused by a streptococcal infection.
   b) Is not seen in adults.
   c) Involves inflammation of the larynx and trachea as far distal as the cricoid cartilage.
   d) Is usually associated with signs of systemic toxaemia.
   e) Should be treated by urgent tracheostomy and IPPV.

31. Amethocaine:
   a) Is an amide type of local anaesthetic drug.
   b) Is not suitable for epidural or subarachnoid use.
   c) Is effective when applied topically to mucous membranes and skin.
   d) Is associated with the lowest incidence of anaphylactoid reactions of all the local anaesthetics.
   e) Is metabolized in the liver.

32. The spinal canal:
   a) Is narrowest in the lumbar region.
   b) Is limited anteriorly by the anterior longitudinal ligament.
   c) The dura stops at L1/L2.
   d) Contains a network of veins which drain into the azygous system.
   e) May be cannulated through the sacrococcygeal membrane.

33. Verapamil:
   a) Causes atrioventricular conduction block.
   b) Antagonizes the effects of neuromuscular blockers.
   c) May be potentiated by volatile anaesthetics.
   d) Should be stopped 2 weeks prior to elective surgery.
   e) Is a potent anti-dysrhythmic drug.

34. After head injury the maintenance of cerebral perfusion pressure (CPP):
   a) Often improves in response to hyperventilation.
   b) Precludes the use of IPPV and PEEP.
   c) Cannot be measured accurately and requires the use of clinical signs for assessment.
   d) Should be maintained above 40 mmHg.
   e) May require a laparotomy.

35. During performance of a lumbar epidural injection by the midline approach the following structures are traversed by the epidural needle:
   a) Supraspinous ligament.
   b) Anterior longitudinal ligament.
   c) Ligamentum flavum.
   d) Dura mater.
   e) Posterior longitudinal ligament.

36. Features which have a positive correlation with postoperative nausea and vomiting include:
   a) Age >70 years.
   b) Obesity.
   c) Female gender.
   d) A history of motion sickness.
   e) Age <3 years.

37. The brachial plexus:
   a) Comprises the posterior primary rami of nerve roots C5 to T1.
   b) Crosses the first rib between scalenus anterior and scalenus medius.
   c) Gives rise to the median and ulnar nerves from its medial cord.
   d) Is closely applied to the subclavian vein.
   e) Is surrounded by a fascial sheath.

38. Causes of vitamin B_{12} deficiency include:
a) Pernicious anaemia.
b) Coeliac disease.
c) Alcohol.
d) Resection of the terminal ileum.
e) Folate deficiency.

39. Features of severe hypokalaemia include:
a) U waves.
b) Tall peaked T waves.
c) Supraventricular ectopic beats.
d) Ventricular ectopic beats.
e) A prolonged QT interval.

40. Compared with the non-pregnant state, changes which are seen in the third trimester include:
a) An increase in cardiac output of 5–10%.
b) An increase in stroke volume.
c) A fall in heart rate.
d) An increase in peripheral vascular resistance.
e) A fall in mean arterial blood pressure.

41. Activated charcoal:
a) Has a large surface area, in the region of $1000\,m^2/g$.
b) Irreversibly binds a large number of drugs.
c) Does not bind highly ionized compounds.
d) Is recommended in repeated doses for poisoning with theophyllines, salicylates and carbamazepine.
e) Often causes nausea and vomiting.

42. Autonomic neuropathy causes:
a) Diarrhoea.
b) Vomiting.
c) A pronounced response to the Valsalva manoeuvre.
d) Proteinuria.
e) Loss of sinus arrhythmia.

43. In diabetic ketoacidosis:
a) Hartmann's solution (Ringer's lactate) can be used after the correction of plasma glucose.
b) The primary action of insulin in lowering plasma glucose is by decreasing hepatic gluconeogenesis rather than peripheral utilization of glucose.
c) Abdominal pain may be the presenting complaint.
d) There is a profound metabolic and respiratory acidosis.
e) There is a high anion gap.

44. Non-insulin-dependent diabetics undergoing surgery:
a) Are not at risk of hypoglycaemia.
b) Experience a more pronounced hyperglycaemic and catabolic response to surgery than insulin-dependent diabetics.
c) There is no autonomic neuropathy.
d) Require less insulin than insulin-dependent diabetics.
e) Do not become ketotic.

45. In rheumatoid arthritis:
a) The cervical spine is involved in 80% of patients.
b) There is an increased blood volume.
c) The majority of cases of atlanto-axial subluxation are asymptomatic.
d) In the absence of other lung disease, an obstructive pattern is often seen in respiratory function tests.
e) There is no association with valvular heart disease.

46. In patients with congestive cardiac failure:
a) The most common cause in the developed world is ischaemic heart disease.
b) Coronary blood flow, oxygen supply and removal of metabolites may be normal.
c) Nitrates act by decreasing afterload and increasing cardiac output.
d) Angiotensin converting enzyme inhibitors cause arterial and venous dilatation.
e) Proteinuria (0.5–1.5 g/day) indicates coincident renal disease.

47. Acute tubular necrosis is characterized by:
a) Urinary osmolality > plasma osmolality.
b) Increased urine:plasma ratio for urea.
c) Increased urine:plasma ratio for creatinine.
d) Oliguria.
e) Elevated urinary sodium.

48. In glucose-6-phosphate dehydrogenase deficiency:
a) There is haemolysis and methaemoglobinaemia due to lack of reduced glutathione.
b) The methaemoglobinaemia responds to methylene blue.
c) Haemolysis may be caused by sulphonamides, chloroquine, prilocaine and tolbutamide.
d) The pentose phosphate pathway is blocked.
e) Vitamin C and vitamin K cause haemolysis.

49. Concerning pulse oximetry:
a) The isobestic point for oxyhaemoglobin and reduced haemoglobin is 650 nm.
b) The maximum difference between the absorption spectra of oxyhaemoglobin and reduced haemoglobin is at 800 nm.
c) The difference between the absorption value at 650 nm and that at 800 nm is proportional to the degree of oxygenation.
d) Lambert's Law states that absorbence of incident light is proportional to the thickness of the absorbing layer.
e) Beer's Law states that absorbence is proportional to the concentration of the molecule absorbing light.

50. Concerning blood gases:
a) The 'standard bicarbonate' is the plasma concentration of bicarbonate ion in fully oxygenated blood at 37°C which has been equilibrated with a gas having a pCO_2 of 5.3 kPa.
b) The 'actual bicarbonate' is the amount of bicarbonate present in plasma at a pCO_2 of 5.3 kPa.
c) The 'base excess' is the amount of strong acid or base required to titrate a litre of blood to a pH of 7.4 at a pCO_2 of 5.3 kPa.
d) Base deficit is a negative base excess.
e) The 'standard base excess' assumes a haemoglobin concentration of 5 g per 100 ml.

51. One Newton equals:
   a) $1 \ Pa \, m^{-2}$.
   b) $1 \ J \, m^{-1}$.
   c) $1 \ kg \, m^{-1} \, s^2$.
   d) $1 \ kg \, m \ s^{-2}$.
   e) $1 \ W \, m^{-1} \, s$.

52. In a supine patient:
   a) The manubriosternal angle is the surface marking of the right atrium.
   b) Use of the manubriosternal angle as the zero for central venous pressure measurement will often produce a negative value.
   c) The right atrium lies in a coronal plane midway between the xiphisternum and the dorsum of the body of the patient.
   d) The right atrium lies in a coronal plane at the mid-axillary line.
   e) The manubriosternal junction is higher than the right atrium.

53. When a peripheral nerve stimulator is used:
   a) The common electrode is proximal.
   b) On the ulnar nerve, both electrodes should be placed as far distal as possible to avoid stimulation of flexor carpi ulnaris and flexor digitorum profundis.
   c) The output waveform of the nerve stimulator should be rectangular.
   d) The optimal length of the pulse current is 0.2 ms.
   e) Neural function is a direct function of the current density applied to the nerve.

54. Bacterial endocarditis:
   a) Will not occur in structurally normal hearts.
   b) The mitral valve is affected more often than the aortic valve.
   c) Is usually streptococcal and sensitive to amoxycillin.
   d) Staphylococcal bacterial endocarditis is usually resistant to amoxycillin.
   e) Patients with previous rheumatic fever, fully treated with penicillin at the time, are not at increased risk of endocarditis compared with normal patients.

55. The following coagulation factors are serine proteases:
   a) II, VII, IX, X.
   b) IX, XI, XII.
   c) V.
   d) IV.
   e) VIII.

56. During pregnancy:
   a) There is an increase in blood volume of 30–40%.
   b) The haematocrit decreases.
   c) There is an increase in red cell 2,3-diphosphoglycerate.
   d) The P_{50} of the oxygen–haemoglobin dissociation curve is decreased.
   e) There is a fall in colloid oncotic pressure.

57. The anion gap:
   a) Exists because the sum of measured anions (chloride and bicarbonate) exceeds the sum of the measured cations.
   b) Is normally 10–14 mmol/l.
   c) Is increased whenever there is a metabolic acidosis.
   d) May be normal in metabolic acidosis if there is a compensatory hyperchloraemia.
   e) Is normal in diabetic ketoacidosis.

58. Effects of intravenous sodium bicarbonate (8.4%) include:
   a) Hypertonicity and hyperosmolality.
   b) Arterial and venous hypercapnia.
   c) Intracellular acidosis.
   d) A low ionized calcium concentration.
   e) Rebound acidosis.

59. Cardiac effects of hypothermia include:
   a) Bradycardia.
   b) Ventricular fibrillation.
   c) J waves on the ECG.
   d) Atrial fibrillation.
   e) A fall in cardiac output in response to reduced tissue oxygen requirements.

60. Variance:

a) Is the sum of the squared deviations from the mean divided by the number of observations.

b) Is the sum of the standard deviations from the mean divided by the number of observations.

c) Is the square root of the standard deviation.

d) Is the square of the standard deviation.

e) Is the standard deviation divided by the square root of the degrees of freedom.

Exam no. 1   Answers

1. a) True.
   b) False. It increases.
   c) False. It is the actual mass of water present in a given
      volume of air.
   d) True.
   e) True.

2. a) True.
   b) True.
   c) True.
   d) False. Pressure or potential energy falls at this point because
      speed or kinetic energy has increased and the total
      energy in the system remains constant.
   e) False. Liquids too, as seen in some nebulizers.

3. a) True.   Since it uses only two wavelengths of light, a pulse oximeter can only differentiate between two kinds of haemoglobin: oxyhaemoglobin and deoxyhaemoglobin. Any other compounds which absorb light from the oximeter will contribute to the pulse-added absorbence signal and will be interpreted as being one of these compounds or a combination of the two. Carboxyhaemoglobin has a pattern of absorption at 660 nm and 940 nm which is interpreted by the oximeter as indicating the presence of oxyhaemoglobin and a high SpO_2 value is produced. If there is a clinical suspicion of the presence of carboxyhaemoglobinaemia, a co-oximeter should be used to determine its presence and concentration.

b) True.   In the presence of methaemoglobin, the pattern of light absorption makes the SpO_2 value produced tend towards 85% irrespective of the true value.

c) False. The light extinction coefficients of HbF, at the relevant wavelengths, are similar to those of HbA and so readings should be accurate in neonates.

d) True.   Deep jaundice may be a cause of falsely low readings.

e) True.   Methylene blue produces large falls in the SpO_2 reading shortly after administration, which last for several minutes. This is important because this dye is often used in the treatment of methaemoglobinaemia.
Saidman and Smith, *Monitoring in Anaesthesia*, (1993) Butterworth Heinemann, pp. 12–19.

4. a) True.
  b) True.
  c) False.
  d) False.
  e) False.

5. a) False. Ten.
  b) False. These are the bipolar leads.
  c) True.
  d) True.
  e) True.

6. a) True. Amino acid.
   b) True. Amine.
   c) True. Peptide.
   d) True.
   e) False.

7. a) False. Anterior pituitary.
   b) False. Polypeptide.
   c) True.
   d) False. Inhibited. Dopamine is the physiological prolactin-inhibiting hormone secreted into the portal hypophyseal vessels.
   e) False. Stimulates and is necessary for lactation to occur.

8. a) False. Secreted by the anterior pituitary.
   b) True.
   c) True.
   d) True.
   e) True.

9. a) False. Mean arterial blood pressure of <90 mmHg.
   b) True. This increases the hydrostatic pressure within the tubules and reduces the gradient across the glomerular membrane.
   c) True. Reduces the surface area available for filtration.
   d) False. Mannitol tends to increase the osmotic pressure of the glomerular filtrate, bringing it nearer to that of the plasma, and reduces the difference due to the oncotic pressure of the plasma proteins.
   e) True.

10. a) True.
    b) True. Not all the urea filtered is excreted.
    c) True.
    d) True.
    e) False. The basis of the accurate measurement of GFR.

11. a) True.
   b) False.
   c) False.
   d) True. This reflects the greater affinity of HbF than HbA for oxygen, allowing transfer of oxygen from maternal haemoglobin to fetal haemoglobin.
   e) True. 2,3-DPG increases the P_{50} of haemoglobin and so increases oxygen delivery to tissues. It is increased in a number of circumstances, including anaemia and chronic hypoxia.

12. a) False. 0.75–1.5 mmol/l.
   b) True.
   c) True.
   d) False. Magnesium ions inhibit the entry of Ca^{2+} ions into nerve terminals.
   e) False.

13. a) True.
   b) True.
   c) False. Factor VIII acts only in the intrinsic pathway.
   d) False. The activator of the extrinsic system.
   e) False. Protein C acts to limit the extent of coagulation by inactivating the activated forms of factors V and VIII.

14. a) False. Renal blood flow is measured by para-amino hippuric acid clearance since it is cleared completely from plasma by the kidneys. Inulin is used to measure glomerular filtration rate.
   b) True.
   c) False. Most of the renal blood flow is directed to the cortex.
   d) False. In health, renal blood flow is autoregulated between mean systolic pressures of 80–180 mmHg.
   e) False. The NSAIDs inhibit local renal prostaglandin synthesis and, hence, renal blood flow, even in normal subjects. In hypovolaemia, this effect may produce an episode of acute renal failure.

15. a) True. Right-to-left shunt is an important contributor to the
$(A-a)$ pO_2 difference. Deoxygenated blood passes from
the right to the left circulation and lowers the arterial
pO_2. The larger the shunt the more difficult it becomes
to restore the arterial pO_2 by increasing the F_IO_2.
b) True.
c) False. This is a determinant of the amount of CO_2 expired
but has no influence on the $(A-a)$ pO_2 gradient.
d) True. By influencing the mixed venous pO_2, cardiac output
affects the magnitude of the $(A-a)$ pO_2 gradient.
e) True. Anaemia tends to increase the $(A-a)$ pO_2 gradient.

16. a) True. Including catecholamines and 5-hydroxytryptamine.
b) False. Steroid hormones interact with receptors distant from
their site of synthesis.
c) True. These are multiple in the CNS and include substance P
and endogenous opioids.
d) True. Gamma amino butyric acid and glycine are examples
of these.
e) True.

17. a) True.
b) False.
c) True.
d) True.
e) False.

18. a) True. Although better against Gram negative infections, this
group have a useful action against Gram positive
organisms, especially *Staphylococcus aureus*. They
have a limited effect against haemolytic streptococci
and pneumococci.
b) False.
c) False. Although nephrotoxic, these drugs may be used in
renal impairment, with monitoring of plasma levels to
ensure efficacy and avoid toxicity.
d) False. These drugs impair calcium release at the
neuromuscular junction.
e) False.

19. a) False. The elimination half-life is shorter at 1.5 h compared with 4 h for fentanyl.
b) True.
c) False.
d) True. A lower pK_a of 6.8 means that 85% of alfentanil is un-ionized at pH 7.4 and this produces a rapid onset of action.
e) True.

20. a) False. Adenosine is a coronary vasodilator and this is the basis of its use in diagnosing coronary artery disease.
b) True.
c) False. Plasma half-life is 1.5 s.
d) False. It is metabolized in erythrocytes and endothelial cells.
e) True.

21. a) False. Heparin is an activator of antithrombin III.
b) False. This is the test to monitor warfarin therapy. Heparin is monitored using the APTT.
c) False. Heparin is the anticoagulant of choice during pregnancy since it does not cross the placenta.
d) True.
e) True.

22. a) False. A synthetic catecholamine.
b) True.
c) False.
d) True.
e) True.

23. a) True. A pharmacodynamic interaction occurs when one drug alters the action of another at its site of action. These two antibiotics act at different points in the bacterial cell wall to produce a synergistic action.
b) True. These affect cardiac conducting tissue and myocardium by different mechanisms to produce the same result.
c) True. Aminoglycosides interfere with calcium flux at the neuromuscular junction and may enhance the effects of non-depolarizing neuromuscular blockers.
d) False. This is a pharmacokinetic interaction where enzyme induction by alcohol produces enhanced metabolism of warfarin.
e) False. This is another pharmacokinetic interaction where diuretics reduce the excretion of lithium.

24. a) False. Aspirin has well proven benefits in the secondary
prevention of cardiac and cerebral infarction and
although there is evidence to support a role in primary
prevention this is not yet a recognized indication for
the drug.

b) False. Aspirin is contraindicated in children younger than 12
years (other than in the treatment of juvenile arthritis)
because of the association with Reye's disease in
febrile children.

c) False. There is very strong evidence to show that aspirin
given in the perioperative period reduces the incidence
of deep venous thrombosis (although it is not widely
used for this purpose). There is no evidence to support
the use of aspirin to treat an established deep venous
thrombosis.

d) True. Several large studies have shown a significant effect of
aspirin in reducing the incidence of reinfarction and
death following myocardial infarction.

e) True.

25. a) True.

b) True.

c) True.

d) True. Opioid receptors exist on the peripheral end of primary
afferent neurons and their activation may directly
decrease neurotransmission or inhibit the release of
excitatory neurotransmitters, such as substance P. There
is clinical evidence in support of a clinical role for
opioids as peripheral analgesics.

e) True. G protein-coupled receptors constitute 80% of known
membrane receptors. They consist of seven peptide
subunits and span cell membranes.

26. a) False. Almost entirely eliminated by hepatic metabolism.

b) True. 96–97%.

c) False.

d) False.

e) True. May cause hypotonia, hypothermia and a withdrawal
syndrome in neonates who are exposed to them
because of maternal use.

27. a) False. Potency decreases – note the high MAC values for desflurane and sevoflurane.
   b) True.
   c) True.
   d) False. MAC decreases in elderly people. It will also be lower in premature and newborn children.
   e) False. The incorporation of fluorine rather than chlorine or bromine tends to reduce blood solubility and increase the speed of uptake and elimination.

28. a) True.
   b) False. Normal blood volume is 75–80 ml/kg. This is excessive.
   c) True. 5–7 mg/kg.
   d) False. Below the age of ten uncuffed tubes are usually used.
   e) False. Epidural analgesia is very useful in paediatric practice, if appropriate expertise and equipment is available.

29. a) True. Full anticoagulation with warfarin and heparin is effective but is not commonly used for obvious reasons.
   b) True. Aspirin has an anti-thrombotic effect because of its actions on platelets. This effect is usually exploited in the prophylaxis of arterial thrombosis but it is also effective in preventing venous thrombosis.
   c) True.
   d) True. Dextran 70 interferes with platelet aggregation. There is a small risk of an anaphylactic reaction.
   e) False. The effects of NSAIDs other than aspirin on platelets are reversible and have not been shown to reduce the incidence of postoperative DVT.

30. a) True.
   b) False.
   c) False.
   d) True.
   e) False.

31. a) True.
   b) False.
   c) True.
   d) False.
   e) True.

32. a) False.
   b) False.
   c) False.
   d) True.
   e) True.

33. a) True.
   b) False.
   c) True.
   d) False.
   e) True.

34. a) True. The CPP is MAP – ICP and hyperventilation often reduces the ICP.
   b) False. After maintenance of a clear airway, adequate oxygenation is a priority.
   c) False. The use of intracranial pressure monitors, such as the Camino transducer, is now common in severe head injuries.
   d) True.
   e) True. To stop haemorrhage which lowers the CPP because of hypotension.

35. a) True.
   b) False. The anterior and posterior longitudinal ligaments unite the vertebral bodies and an epidural needle should never get near them.
   c) True.
   d) False. This is relatively common but not a desired part of the technique.
   e) False.

36. a) False.
   b) True.
   c) True.
   d) True.
   e) False.

37. a) False. Anterior primary rami.
   b) True.
   c) True.   The median nerve also has an origin from the lateral cord.
   d) False. The plexus is separated from the subclavian vein by the scalenus anterior.
   e) True.   This is an extension of the prevertebral fascia which covers the scalenus muscles.

38. a) True.   This autoimmune disease prevents intrinsic factor synthesis and vitamin B_{12} absorption.
   b) True.
   c) False. This produces macrocytosis and may be involved in the aetiology of several kinds of anaemia, e.g. iron deficiency anaemia.
   d) True.   This is the site of absorption of the vitamin B_{12}-intrinsic factor complex and resection or disease here may cause vitamin B_{12} deficiency.
   e) False. This is another cause of megaloblastic anaemia.

39. a) True.   One of the classical features.
   b) False. A classical feature of hyperkalaemia.
   c) True.   Both ventricular and supraventricular dysrhythmias are common.
   d) True.
   e) False. The QT interval is normal in hypokalaemia but may be difficult to measure properly because of small T waves and prominent U waves.

40. a) False. 30–50%.
  b) True.
  c) False. The increase in cardiac output is due to a combination of an increase in heart rate and an increase in stroke volume.
  d) False.
  e) True.

41. a) True. Activated charcoal is charcoal that has been treated in a stream of gas or by chemical activators to increase its surface area.
  b) False. Binding to activated charcoal is reversible.
  c) True. Such as ferrous sulphate, lithium carbonate, strong acids and alkalis, and cyanides.
  d) True. This applies to drugs which are likely to remain unabsorbed in the gut for many hours.
  e) True.

42. a) True.
  b) True. Diminished gastric motility and delayed gastric emptying are common in autonomic neuropathy. Vomiting as a result of this is less common but well recognized.
  c) False. The initial increase in heart rate during forced expiration and the subsequent decrease when the manoeuvre ends are attenuated by an autonomic neuropathy.
  d) False.
  e) True. This can be used as a simple bedside test.

43. a) False   Lactate containing solutions should be avoided.
  b) True.
  c) True.
  d) False.
  e) True.

  Diabetes (1988) **37**: 1470–1477.

44. a) False.
b) True.
c) False.
d) False.
e) False. This can happen during a severe illness.

45. a) True.
b) True.
c) True.
d) False. Restrictive.
e) False. Thickening, inflammation, and granulomata of valve leaflets and ring usually in the aortic or more rarely mitral valves occurs in up to 30% of patients but is rarely of clinical significance. Pericardial inflammation occurs in about 50% of patients but is rarely associated with a significant pericardial effusion.

46. a) True.
b) True.
c) False. These drugs are systemic and pulmonary venodilators. The cardiac output does not usually increase.
d) True.
e) False. This is commonly seen in congestive cardiac failure and resolves when the cardiac output increases.

47. a) False.
b) False.
c) False.
d) True.
e) True.
   Annals of Internal Medicine (1978) **89**: 47–50.

48. a) True.
b) False. Methylene blue may worsen the haemolysis.
c) True.
d) True.
e) True.

49. a) False. 800 nm.
　　b) False. 650 nm.
　　c) True.
　　d) True.
　　e) True.

50. a) True.
　　b) True.
　　c) True.
　　d) True.
　　e) True.
　　　　　Sykes, Vickers and Hull, *Principles of Measurement and Monitoring in Anaesthesia and Intensive Care*, (1991) Third Edition, Blackwell Scientific Publications.

51. a) True.
　　b) True. 1 Joule = 1 N.m.
　　c) False. 1 Pascal
　　d) True.
　　e) True. 1 Watt = $1\,\mathrm{J\,s^{-1}}$.

52. a) False.
　　b) True.
　　c) True.
　　d) False.
　　e) True.
　　　　　Sykes, Vickers and Hull, *Principles of Measurement and Monitoring in Anaesthesia and Intensive Care*, (1991) Third Edition, Blackwell Scientific Publications.

53. a) False. Distal.
　　b) True.
　　c) True.
　　d) True.
　　e) True. Unlike neuromuscular transmission which depends on the degree of neuromuscular blockade.

54. a) False.
   b) False.
   c) True.
   d) True.
   e) False.

55. a) True.
   b) True.
   c) False.
   d) False. This is Ca^{2+}.
   e) False.

56. a) True.
   b) True.
   c) True.
   d) False.
   e) True.

57. a) False. The measured cations (sodium and potassium) exceed the measured anions (chloride and bicarbonate). The anion gap represents unmeasured anions: mostly protein, phosphate and sulphate.
   b) True.
   c) False. It is increased in most metabolic acidoses but not if there is a compensatory hyperchloraemia developed as bicarbonate is lost.
   d) True.
   e) False. This is a condition where the unmeasured anions are markedly increased, e.g. lactate, hydroxybutyrate and pyruvate.

58. a) True.
   b) True.
   c) True.
   d) True.
   e) False. Alkalosis.

59. a) True.
   b) True.
   c) True.
   d) True.
   e) False.

60. a) True.
   b) False.
   c) False.
   d) True.
   e) False. This is the standard error of the mean.

Exam no. 2   Questions

1. **Concerning solubility:**
   a) The amount of gas dissolved in a given volume of liquid falls as the temperature is increased at constant pressure.
   b) Factors which influence the solubility of a gas include partial pressure, temperature and latent heat of vaporization.
   c) Henry's Law states that at a given temperature the amount of a gas dissolved in a given solvent is directly proportional to the partial pressure of gas in equilibrium with the liquid.
   d) The Bunsen solubility coefficient is the volume of gas which dissolves in unit volume of the solvent.
   e) The Ostwald solubility coefficient is the volume of gas which dissolves in unit volume of the solvent at ambient temperature and pressure.

2. **Isotopes of the same element:**
   a) Have the same number of protons.
   b) Have the same number of neutrons.
   c) Have a different electrical charge.
   d) Have the same atomic number.
   e) Have the same atomic weight.

3. **Oxygen:**
   a) Is manufactured by the hydrolysis of steam.
   b) Has a boiling point of −119°C.
   c) Has a molecular weight of 16.
   d) Has an isotope called ozone.
   e) Has a critical temperature of −183°C.

4. **Concerning electricity:**
   a) Impedance is the same as resistance.
   b) A potential difference of 1 V exists between two points when 1 watt of energy is released by the transfer of 1 ampere of electricity between them.
   c) A flow of one ampere for 1 s transfers 1 coulomb of electricity.
   d) Electrical power is expressed in amperes.
   e) An alternating current of 240 V has a peak amplitude of 340 V.

5. **A pulse oximeter is likely to give spurious readings in the presence of:**
   a) Hypothermia.
   b) Anaemia.
   c) Polycythaemia.
   d) Hypotension.
   e) Hypertension.

6. **In a trace of the central venous pressure waveform:**
   a) The mean pressure displayed is relative to the right atrium.
   b) A negative value means that the system is open to air.
   c) The mean pressure is unaffected by the application of PEEP at 5 cm H_2O.
   d) The 'v' wave is caused by atrial contraction.
   e) Placing the patient in the head down position will increase the CVP.

7. **A 40% Ventimask:**
   a) Requires an oxygen flow of 8 l/min.
   b) Is accurate to within 2%.
   c) Acts as an additional dead space.
   d) Will deliver a higher F_iO_2 than 40% if the oxygen flow rate is increased.
   e) Will always deliver an F_iO_2 of 40%.

8. The adrenal cortex:
  a) Produces hormones which are derivatives of cholesterol.
  b) Secretes the mineralocorticoid fludrocortisone.
  c) Secretes the glucocorticoids dexamethasone and cortisol.
  d) Is sensitive to circulating ACTH and angiotensin II which increase glucocorticoid secretion.
  e) Both glucocorticoid and mineralocorticoid secretion are stimulated by metyrapone.

9. Acetylcholine:
  a) Is the acetyl ester of choline.
  b) Is synthesized from choline and acetyl co-enzyme A.
  c) Is hydrolysed by the enzyme choline acetyltransferase.
  d) Is a central neurotransmitter.
  e) May be hydrolysed by pseudocholinesterase.

10. Testosterone:
  a) Is structurally a steroid.
  b) Is synthesized in the Sertoli cells of the testis.
  c) May be synthesized in the adrenal medulla.
  d) Is found in healthy women.
  e) Is mostly protein bound.

11. In a healthy child aged 1 year the following values would be normal:
  a) Weight 9–12 kg.
  b) Heart rate 60–80 beats/min.
  c) Systolic blood pressure 80–110 mmHg.
  d) Respiratory rate 12–16 breaths/min.
  e) Haemoglobin 8–10 g/dl.

12. In the normal kidney:
  a) The proximal and distal tubules secrete hydrogen ions.
  b) Hydrogen ions are buffered by ammonia.
  c) Cortical blood flow is around 4–5 ml/g/min.
  d) Filtered amino acids are not reabsorbed.
  e) The proximal convoluted tubules reabsorb 60–70% of the glomerular filtrate.

13. Fetal haemoglobin:
a) Consists of two alpha and two beta polypeptide chains.
b) Binds 2,3-DPG more avidly than does HbA.
c) Has a lower P_{50} than HbA.
d) Has usually disappeared from the circulation by 4 weeks after birth.
e) Comprises about 80% of the total haemoglobin at birth.

14. The following stimulate platelet aggregation:
a) Mechanical distortion.
b) Collagen.
c) Prostacyclin.
d) Adenosine diphosphate.
e) Lignocaine.

15. Thrombin:
a) Stimulates platelet aggregation.
b) Converts fibrinogen to fibrin.
c) Inactivates antithrombin III.
d) Activates factors V and VIII.
e) Inhibits protein C.

16. The following are components of vital capacity:
a) Residual volume.
b) Closing capacity.
c) Functional residual capacity.
d) Tidal volume.
e) FEV_1.

17. Insulin:
a) Is secreted by the exocrine pancreas.
b) Is secreted as the prohormone proinsulin which is converted to insulin in the plasma.
c) Has a half-life in plasma of 2–4 h.
d) Is metabolized largely in the liver and kidneys.
e) Exerts many of its actions by binding to a specific receptor, which is a tetrameric protein.

18. Systemic effects of interleukin-6 include:
a) Pyrexia.
b) Anorexia.
c) A fall in circulating neutrophils.
d) Inhibition of T and B lymphocytes.
e) Increased prostaglandin synthesis.

19. 5-Hydroxytryptamine:
a) Is found in the central nervous system, intestine and platelets.
b) Is metabolized mainly to 5-hydroxyindoleacetic acid.
c) May be antagonized by ondansetron and methysergide.
d) Is a major inflammatory mediator in the periphery.
e) Is involved in the central processing of nociceptive stimuli.

20. Methoxamine:
a) Is a potent alpha agonist.
b) May cause a tachycardia.
c) Reduces urine output.
d) Is secreted by the adrenal glands.
e) Should not be used in patients receiving halothane.

21. Fentanyl citrate:
a) When given as an intravenous bolus of 2 µg/kg has a duration of action of 20–30 min.
b) Has a volume of distribution in normal adults of 3.7 l/kg.
c) Has a terminal elimination half-life of 1.5 h.
d) Does not cross the placenta.
e) Is contraindicated in patients taking monoamine oxidase inhibitors.

22. Aprotinin:
a) Inhibits platelet aggregation.
b) Is a serine protease inhibitor.
c) Is a thrombotic agent.
d) Is an anticoagulant.
e) Converts inactive plasminogen into active plasmin.

23. The conjugation of drugs with glucuronic acid to form glucuronides:
a) Increases the water solubility of most compounds.
b) Renders the drug inactive.
c) Reduces the rate of urinary excretion.
d) Occurs primarily in the liver.
e) Has limited potential to metabolize drugs in children because of the incomplete maturation of enzyme systems.

24. The following drug interactions occur as a result of pharmacokinetic factors:
a) Morphine and naloxone.
b) Disulfiram and alcohol.
c) Cimetidine and diazepam.
d) Warfarin and vitamin K.
e) Probenicid and penicillin.

25. Concerning the elimination half-life of a drug:
a) It is defined as 50% of the time required to eliminate a drug from the body.
b) It is proportional to volume of distribution and inversely proportional to clearance.
c) It is the only variable which determines the rate at which a drug accumulates in the body during regular multiple-dosing or infusion.
d) In a healthy adult is 2–4 h for morphine sulphate.
e) If it is prolonged, a steady state during infusion will be reached more quickly than normal.

26. The following drugs are dopaminergic antagonists:
a) Metoclopramide.
b) Domperidone.
c) Ondansetron.
d) Prochloperazine.
e) Nabilone.

27. Benzodiazepines:
   a) Act at specific receptor sites in the CNS.
   b) Are antagonists of gamma-amino butyric acid.
   c) Enhance the movement of chloride ions from the intracellular to the extracellular compartments.
   d) Increase the synthesis of gamma-amino butyric acid.
   e) Are naturally present in the CNS.

28. Cytochrome P450 is inhibited by:
   a) Phenytoin.
   b) Rifampicin.
   c) Cimetidine.
   d) Penicillin.
   e) Allopurinol.

29. During laparoscopic cholecystectomy, the production of a pneumoperitoneum may cause:
   a) Endobronchial intubation.
   b) Hypotension.
   c) Metabolic acidosis.
   d) Respiratory acidosis.
   e) Bradycardia.

30. Halothane:
   a) Is a halogenated methyl ethyl ether.
   b) Contains thymol 1% as a preservative.
   c) Should not be used with soda lime.
   d) Is contraindicated in cirrhosis of the liver.
   e) Must not be used more than once in the same patient.

31. The following drugs cross the blood–brain barrier:
   a) Propofol.
   b) Desflurane.
   c) Atropine.
   d) Atracurium.
   e) Glycopyrrolate.

32. Malignant hyperthermia may be triggered by:
a) Bupivacaine.
b) Suxamethonium.
c) Enflurane.
d) Atracurium.
e) Propofol.

33. Phenothiazines:
a) Are effective antiemetics.
b) Have sedative effects.
c) Commonly cause extrapyramidal side effects.
d) May cause cholestatic jaundice.
e) Reduce emesis by binding to 5-HT$_3$ receptors.

34. Tricyclic antidepressants:
a) Must be stopped 3 weeks prior to elective surgery.
b) Have anticholinergic side effects.
c) In overdosage may result in coma and convulsions.
d) Inhibit the pressor response to exogenous catecholamines.
e) Are a contraindication to the use of pethidine.

35. Subarachnoid anaesthesia is contraindicated in patients receiving:
a) Aspirin.
b) Subcutaneous heparin 5000 IU twice daily.
c) Warfarin.
d) Diclofenac sodium.
e) Streptokinase.

36. The femoral nerve:
a) Arises from the posterior divisions of nerve roots L2, L3 and L4.
b) Is a purely motor nerve.
c) Lies between the femoral artery and vein at the groin.
d) Becomes the saphenous nerve distally in the leg.
e) Is blocked as part of a 'three-in-one' block.

37. Recognized complications of nasotracheal intubation include:
a) Dental damage.
b) Lingual nerve palsy.
c) Recurrent laryngeal nerve damage.
d) Sinusitis.
e) Subglottic stenosis.

38. Nitric oxide (NO):
a) Is a physiological vasodilator.
b) Has a half-life of 5 s.
c) Is one of the causes of hypotension in sepsis.
d) Acts via protein kinases.
e) Has metabolites which are excreted by the kidneys.

39. Features of an iron deficiency anaemia may include:
a) Breathlessness.
b) Angina.
c) Jaundice.
d) Peripheral neuropathy.
e) Brittle hair and nails.

40. A serum potassium concentration of 2.7 mmol/l is likely to produce:
a) Motor paralysis.
b) Ventricular ectopic beats.
c) Tetany.
d) Fits.
e) Ileus.

41. If a 55-year-old woman collapses 24 h after an abdominal hysterectomy, the following support a diagnosis of pulmonary embolism:
a) Hypotension.
b) Chest pain.
c) Cyanosis.
d) Abdominal pain.
e) Low jugular venous pressure.

42. Bier's block (intravenous regional anaesthesia):
a) May be performed using any of the local anaesthetics.
b) Is suitable for reduction of Colles fractures.
c) Does not require the patient to be fasted.
d) Provides analgesia lasting into the postoperative period.
e) Has been performed with pethidine and with ketamine.

43. Carcinoma of the prostate:
a) Histologically is a transitional cell tumour.
b) Is usually clinically aggressive and invasive.
c) Produces similar symptoms to benign prostatic hyperplasia.
d) Requires orchidectomy.
e) Is often treated with cyproterone acetate in patients too frail to undergo surgery.

44. In the syndrome of inappropriate ADH secretion:
a) There is continuing ADH secretion despite hypotonicity and a normal or expanded extracellular fluid volume.
b) Diagnosis is made when urinary osmolality exceeds that of the plasma.
c) Mannitol causes ADH secretion and thirst.
d) The condition may be differentiated from sodium depletion by measuring the urinary sodium excretion.
e) Lithium carbonate antagonizes the effects of ADH on the distal tubule.

45. Concerning arterial hypertension:
a) Baroreceptor sensitivity declines with age.
b) Sufferers show an exaggeration of normal variability in blood pressure.
c) Hypertensive smokers suffer twice the incidence of cardiac and cerebrovascular complications of hypertensive non-smokers.
d) Prognosis correlates with the arterial pressure.
e) Baroreceptor sensitivity declines with increased resting mean arterial pressure.

46. When measuring the blood pressure with a manual sphygmomanometer:
a) The cuff width should be half the circumference of the arm.
b) The cuff should be at heart level.
c) Arm position influences the measured blood pressure.
d) The systolic blood pressure tends to be underestimated.
e) The diastolic pressure tends to be overestimated.

47. In haemophilia A:
a) There is X-linked recessive inheritance.
b) The bleeding time is prolonged.
c) Coagulation tests of the intrinsic pathway are prolonged.
d) There is a deficiency of factor VIII.
e) There is a deficiency of factor IX.

48. The anion gap is increased if metabolic acidosis is caused by:
a) Diabetic ketoacidosis.
b) Lactate.
c) Diarrhoea.
d) Pancreatic fistulae.
e) Uraemia.

49. The following are SI units:
a) Metre.
b) Gram.
c) Centigrade.
d) Candela.
e) Ampere.

50. When using electroencephalography:
a) Measured voltages are usually in the range 10–100 µV.
b) Voltages up to 500 µV may be seen during an epileptic fit.
c) Beta waves are abolished by sedatives.
d) Delta waves are normal during sleep.
e) Theta waves occur at a frequency of 4–7 Hz.

51. When performing a lumbar puncture:
a) CSF pressure should be measured in the lateral position with reference to the right atrium.
b) The glucose concentration should be 60–80% of the patient's plasma glucose.
c) Conjugated and unconjugated bilirubin are seen in the CSF of jaundiced patients.
d) A normal CSF pressure is 5–20 mm of CSF.
e) The CSF pressure is elevated in congestive cardiac failure.

52. In beta thalassaemia major:
a) There are decreased alpha and increased beta chains.
b) Only heterozygotes survive childhood.
c) Red cell survival time is normal.
d) There is splenomegaly because of increased splenic erythropoiesis.
e) There is an increase in circulating volume.

53. Neurofibromatosis is associated with:
a) Fibrosing alveolitis.
b) Phaeochromocytoma.
c) Renal artery stenosis.
d) Acoustic neuroma.
e) Epilepsy.

54. Concerning myocardial infarction:
a) ST segment changes precede wall motion abnormalities.
b) Right bundle branch block does not obscure the changes of inferior infarction.
c) ST elevation and subsequent T wave changes can be seen despite left bundle branch block.
d) During diastole ischaemic tissue is more electropositive than surrounding myocardium.
e) Asymmetrical T wave inversion is usually seen over the ensuing 2–3 weeks.

55. Von Willebrand's factor:
a) Is coagulation factor VIII.
b) Links platelets to damaged epithelium.
c) Is released by intravenous DDAVP (desmopressin).
d) When deficient, results in prolongation of the activated partial thromboplastin time.
e) Is protected from destruction when in combination with factor VIII.

56. Thoracic epidural analgesia:
a) Produces intercostal muscle weakness and significantly impairs respiratory function.
b) Increases the duration of a postoperative ileus.
c) After major abdominal surgery, is associated with less radiological evidence of pulmonary morbidity than opioid analgesia.
d) Does not affect diaphragmatic function.
e) After major abdominal surgery, is associated with a reduction in the frequency and severity of episodic hypoxic episodes than opioid analgesia.

57. In poisoning with organophosphate insecticides:
a) The enzyme acetylcholinesterase is irreversibly inhibited.
b) Atropine is indicated for the treatment of muscarinic effects.
c) Effects may follow transdermal absorption.
d) Pralidoxime is therapeutic because it antagonizes acetylcholine at receptors.
e) There is a deficiency of acetylcholine at the neuromuscular junction.

58. Indications for sodium bicarbonate in cardiac arrest include:
a) Metabolic acidosis after a prolonged cardiac arrest.
b) Hyperkalaemia.
c) Low plasma bicarbonate.
d) A pre-existing (pre-arrest) metabolic acidosis.
e) An attempt to lower the defibrillation threshold.

59. In statistics:
   a) APGAR scores are an example of interval data.
   b) The American Society of Anesthesiologists physical status score (ASA I-V) is an example of ordinal data.
   c) $P < 0.05$ means there is a 1-in-200 probability that the findings were purely due to chance.
   d) 95% confidence limits include all values within 2 standard deviations of the mean.
   e) $P > 0.05$ means that the findings are significant to a 1-in-20 level of significance.

60. A screening test for a disease is useful when:
   a) The disease is not rare.
   b) Presymptomatic diagnosis improves the outcome of treatment.
   c) The disease is serious.
   d) The disease is treatable.
   e) Every subject has the disease.

Exam no. 2   Answers

1. a) True.
   b) False. The latent heat of vaporization is irrelevant. The important factors are temperature, partial pressure and the liquid and gas concerned.
   c) True.
   d) False. The Bunsen coefficient requires correction to STP and a partial pressure of gas above the liquid of 1 atmosphere.
   e) True. The Ostwald coefficient has the advantage of being independent of pressure.

2. a) True. This is the definition of an element – molecules with the same number of protons are the same element.
   b) False. Molecules with the same number of protons but different numbers of neutrons are isotopes of the same element.
   c) False. They will all be neutral unless ionized.
   d) True. This is the number of protons found in an atom of each molecule and defines the position of the element in the Periodic Table.
   e) False.

3. a) False. Oxygen is manufactured by the fractional distillation of liquid air after removal of carbon dioxide. It has a boiling point of −183°C while that of nitrogen is −195°C.
   b) False. This the critical temperature above which the gas cannot be liquefied.
   c) False. The atomic number of oxygen is 16 but its molecular weight is 32.
   d) True.
   e) False. This is the boiling point.

4. a) False. Impedance is the term used when there is a dependence on the frequency of the current involved. It is also expressed in Ohms.

   b) True.   This is the definition of a volt.

   c) True.   This is the definition of a Coulomb. It is the equivalent of 6.24×10^{18} electrons.

   d) False. Watts. $1\,W = 1\,J/s$.

   e) True.   The magnitude of an alternating current is expressed as the direct current which would produce an equivalent heating effect. The figure used is the root mean square value, i.e. the square root of the mean of the squared values for the alternating current. The peak value of a 240 V alternating current is 340 V.

5. a) True.   In the presence of profound peripheral vasoconstriction, there is often inadequate peripheral perfusion to give an accurate oximeter reading. Alternatively, there may be peripheral cyanosis in hypothermia which does not reflect the central SaO_2.

   b) False. At low haemoglobin concentrations, a low arterial pO_2 is likely to produce higher values for SpO_2 than if the haemoglobin were normal. However, they are still accurate values for the SpO_2.

   c) False. The reverse is the case in polycythaemia with cyanosis and low SpO_2 readings seen at a normal arterial pO_2.

   d) True.

   e) False. There is no reason why this should be the case.

6. a) False. The mean pressure displayed is relative to the transducer. This is usually placed at the level of the right atrium and, if not, meaningless or misleading information will be displayed.

   b) False. A negative value is quite possible when the patient is hypovolaemic or head up, as well as when the transducer is incorrectly positioned.

   c) False. The exact effect of this will depend on a number of factors, especially lung compliance, but in most cases it will tend to increase the mean CVP reading displayed.

   d) False. This is caused by filling of the right atrium before opening of the tricuspid valve at the end of systole.

   e) True.

7. a) True. The required oxygen flow rate is engraved on the valves which come with the masks.
   b) True.
   c) False. The high fresh gas flow flushes expired gases out of the mask and rebreathing does not occur in normal use. If there were no oxygen being delivered to the mask, or if the flow rate were lower than recommended, rebreathing might occur.
   d) False. The F_iO_2 would remain the same since the entrainment ratio of the valve is fixed. The fresh gas flow to the patient would be increased.
   e) False. Not if the patient's peak inspiratory flow rate exceeds the fresh gas flow rate. This may happen during hyperventilation when air would be entrained.

8. a) True.
   b) False. This is a synthetic mineralocorticoid. The naturally occurring compound is aldosterone.
   c) False. Dexamethasone is a synthetic compound.
   d) False. Angiotensin II stimulates the secretion of aldosterone.
   e) False. This compound is an inhibitor of the adrenal enzyme 11-beta hydroxylase and decreases steroid production.

9. a) True.
   b) True. This reaction is catalysed by the enzyme choline acetyltransferase.
   c) False. Acetylcholinesterase.
   d) True.
   e) True.

10. a) True.
   b) False. Leydig cells.
   c) False. Adrenal cortex.
   d) True. In low concentrations. Synthesized in the ovaries and possibly the adrenals.
   e) True. 98%.

11. a) True.
   b) False. 80–110 beats/min.
   c) True.
   d) False. 20–24.
   e) False.

12. a) True.
   b) True. Other buffers in the tubular fluid include bicarbonate and hydrogen phosphate.
   c) True. Renal cortical blood flow is much higher than medullary flow which varies between 0.03 and 0.2 ml/g/min.
   d) False.
   e) True.

13. a) False. This is the structure of HbA. In HbF, the beta chains are replaced by gamma chains.
   b) False.
   c) True. The higher affinity of HbF for oxygen, compared with HbA, is due to reduced binding of 2,3-DPG by the gamma polypeptide chains.
   d) False. Four months.
   e) True.

14. a) True.
   b) True.
   c) False. This is produced by vascular endothelium as an inhibitor of platelet aggregation.
   d) True. This is released by activated platelets to recruit further platelets to the site of injury.
   e) False. Local anaesthetics have been shown to inhibit platelet aggregation *in vivo* and *in vitro*.

15. a) True. Thrombin has a multitude of actions in the coagulation cascade. As well as its primary action of producing fibrin from fibrinogen, it has a feedback action to increase the amounts of factors V and VIII activated, to enhance platelet aggregation and, along with fibrin, activate factor XIII. As the coagulation cascade is activated, steps to limit its extent must be taken and this includes the activation of several anticoagulant systems including antithrombin III, protein C, protein S and the fibrinolytic system. Thrombin is involved in the activation of these pathways too.
   b) True.
   c) False.
   d) True.
   e) False.

16. a) False. The vital capacity comprises tidal volume, inspiratory reserve volume and expiratory reserve volume.
   b) False. Closing volume comprises residual volume and a variable volume above this and is not a component of vital capacity.
   c) False. FRC also includes the residual volume.
   d) True.
   e) False. FEV_1 is an effort-dependent value and is not part of the vital capacity.

17. a) False. Endocrine.
   b) False. This reaction takes place in the cells of the islands of Langerhans prior to secretion and yields insulin and protein C, which can be assayed. Proinsulin is secreted in unmodified form from islet cell tumours.
   c) False. Five minutes.
   d) True.
   e) True.

18. a) True.
   b) True.
   c) False. Increase.
   d) False. Stimulation.
   e) True.

19. a) True.
   b) True.
   c) True.
   d) True.
   e) True.
   British Journal of Anaesthesia (1994) **73**: 395–407.

20. a) True.
   b) False. By increasing systemic vascular resistance, methoxamine may induce a reflex bradycardia.
   c) True. Methoxamine constricts the renal arteries and reduces GFR.
   d) False. Methoxamine is a synthetic compound.
   e) False.

21. a) True.
   b) True.
   c) False.
   d) False.
   e) True. Fentanyl is structurally similar to pethidine.

22. a) True.
b) True.
c) False. Although aprotinin inhibits fibrinolysis, it is not recognized as having a procoagulant action.
d) True. In the concentrations reached during high dose infusion regimens, aprotinin is an inhibitor of the intrinsic clotting system.
e) False. It inactivates free plasmin.

23. a) True. Many drugs would be very poorly excreted by the kidneys if they were not rendered water-soluble first.
b) False. In many cases, the glucuronides retain activity, e.g. opioids.
c) False. The conjugation is usually necessary to promote urinary excretion.
d) True.
e) False. Children have fully mature enzyme systems for drug metabolism from the age of 4–6 months. In neonates and infants below this age, there will be a limited capacity to metabolize many drugs.

24. a) False. A pharmacokinetic interaction occurs when the absorption, distribution, metabolism or excretion of one drug is altered by the presence of another. The interaction of opioids and naloxone occurs at receptor level and is not pharmacokinetic in nature.
b) True. Disulfiram inhibits the metabolism of acetaldehyde which is a product of ethanol metabolism. This accumulates and causes unpleasant symptoms including flushing, dizziness and diarrhoea. This interaction is the basis of the use of disulfiram in the treatment of alcohol abuse.
c) True. Cimetidine inhibits the metabolism of diazepam by inhibiting cytochrome P450.
d) False. This is an interaction based on antagonism at enzyme level.
e) True. Probenecid competes with penicillin for renal tubular secretory mechanisms so that plasma levels of penicillin are raised and its actions prolonged.

25. a) False.   The elimination half-life of a compound is the time taken for its concentration to halve irrespective of the starting concentration.
   b) True.
   c) True.   Half-life is the only variable affecting the rate of attainment of a steady plasma concentration during infusion or multiple dosing. The dose affects the magnitude of the steady plasma concentration achieved.
   d) True.
   e) False.   If the elimination half-life is prolonged, an infusion will take longer than normal to achieve a steady state and the magnitude of this, when reached, will be higher than if the half-life were normal.

26. a) True.
   b) True.
   c) False.   Ondansetron is a specific antagonist of serotonin ($5HT_3$).
   d) True.   The phenothiazines exert their antiemetic action by several mechanisms, including antidopaminergic and antihistaminergic.
   e) False.   This is a synthetic cannabinoid which probably acts on specific receptors.

27. a) True.   Found on the α-subunits of the GABA receptors.
   b) False.
   c) False.   Extracellular to intracellular, leading to cellular hyperpolarization and reduced excitability.
   d) False.
   e) True.   Found in small amounts in synaptic vesicles and are thought to play a role in memory.

28. a) False.
   b) False.
   c) True.
   d) False.
   e) True.

29. a) True. Displacement of the diaphragm cephalad reduces lung
volumes and may reduce compliance and cause
endobronchial intubation.

b) True. A reduction in venous return, along with the head-up
position, reduces cardiac output which may cause
hypotension and, during a prolonged procedure,
metabolic acidosis.

c) True.

d) True. Absorption of carbon dioxide along with possible
hypoventilation as a result of a fall in lung compliance
may produce hypercarbia unless a capnograph is used.

e) True. A bradycardia or a tachycardia may be seen
particularly when the head up position is assumed.

30. a) False.
b) False. 0.01%.
c) False.
d) False.
e) False.

31. a) True.
b) True.
c) True.
d) False.
e) False.

32. a) False.
b) True.
c) True.
d) False.
e) False.

33. a) True.
b) True.
c) False.
d) True.
e) False.

34. a) False.
  b) True.
  c) True.
  d) False.
  e) False.

35. a) False.
  b) False.
  c) True.   There is general agreement that anticoagulation and thrombolysis are almost complete contraindications to subarachnoid and epidural anaesthesia because of the perceived risk of an epidural haematoma. Patients taking NSAIDs and subcutaneous heparin commonly present for surgery and there is no evidence that central neural blockade in these circumstances is harmful.
  d) False.
  e) True.

36. a) True.
  b) False. It is a mixed motor and sensory nerve.
  c) False. Lateral to the artery.
  d) True.
  e) True. This will block the femoral, obturator and lateral cutaneous nerves.

37. a) True. This is usually caused by laryngoscopy rather than intubation.
  b) False. This may occur during orotracheal intubation.
  c) True. This is usually due to pressure of the inflated cuff on the laminae of the thyroid cartilage. The lesion is usually unilateral and temporary, producing a change in voice.
  d) True. This is particularly common during long term intubation in intensive care units and is one reason why this route is rarely used, at least in adult units.
  e) True. This is a complication of prolonged intubation by either route. It is a particular problem in children but can occur in adults.

38. a) True.
    b) True.
    c) True.
    d) True.
    e) True.

39. a) True. This will occur in any anaemia if it is severe enough, as will angina.
    b) True.
    c) False. A feature of severe haemolysis.
    d) False. Seen in vitamin B_{12} deficiency.
    e) True.

40. a) False. This is described in severe hypokalaemia but is unlikely at this level of serum potassium.
    b) True. Both atrial and ventricular dysrhythmias commonly occur and sudden ventricular fibrillation is common.
    c) False. Tetany is a feature of hypocalcaemia, as are fits.
    d) False.
    e) True. An ileus is one of the commonest manifestations of hypokalaemia, especially in surgical patients.

41. a) True.
    b) True.
    c) True.
    d) False.
    e) False. With a large embolus this will be high.

42. a) False.
    b) True.
    c) False.
    d) False.
    e) True.

43. a) False. Adenocarcinoma
 b) False. This tends to be an indolent tumour with a long natural history. Up to 30% of asymptomatic men are found to have foci of malignancy at autopsy.
 c) True.
 d) False. Prostatic carcinoma and its metastases are androgen-dependent and orchidectomy may be performed to encourage remission of metastases by removing the main source of androgens.
 e) False. This steroid hormone exerts an anti-androgen effect and is used to encourage remission of these tumours and their metastases, usually as an adjunct to surgery rather than in place of it.

44. a) True.
 b) False. Evidence of volume expansion is also required.
 c) True. Mannitol cannot enter osmoreceptor cells thereby creating an osmotic gradient and stimulating ADH release.
 d) True. With normal renal function, in sodium depletion the urinary sodium is low (<20 mmol/l) while with SIADH the urinary sodium is >20 mmol/l.
 e) True.

45. a) True.
 b) True.
 c) True.
 d) True.
 e) True.

46. a) True.
 b) True.
 c) True.
 d) True.
 e) True.

47. a) True.
   b) False.
   c) True.
   d) True.
   e) False. This is haemophilia B.

48. a) True.
   b) True.
   c) False. The anion gap does not increase in metabolic acidosis due to bicarbonate loss because of compensatory hyperchloraemia.
   d) False.
   e) True.

49. a) True. The SI units are metre, second, kilogram, ampere, Kelvin, mole and candela.
   b) False.
   c) False.
   d) True.
   e) True.

50. a) True.
   b) True.
   c) False. Enhanced.
   d) True.
   e) True.

51. a) True.
   b) True.
   c) True.
   d) False. Centimetres.
   e) True.

52. a) False. Absent or decreased beta chains and increased alpha
           chains.
       b) False.
       c) False. Reduced because of precipitation of alpha chains in
           erythrocytes.
       d) False. Increased red cell destruction in the spleen.
       e) True. Increased because of splenomegaly and bone marrow
           expansion.

53. a) True.
       b) True.
       c) True.
       d) True.
       e) True.

54. a) False.
       b) True.
       c) True.
       d) True.
       e) False. Symmetrical.

55. a) False.
       b) True.
       c) True.
       d) False.
       e) False. von Willebrand's factor protects factor VIII from
           destruction.

56. a) False.
       b) False.
       c) True.
       d) True.
       e) True.

Anesthesiology (1995) **52**: 1474–1506.

57. a) True.
  b) True.
  c) True.
  d) False. It regenerates active acetylcholinesterase.
  e) False. Excess.

58. a) True.
  b) True.
  c) False.
  d) True.
  e) False.

59. a) False. APGAR scores are ordinal data.
  b) True. ASA scores are rankings not measurements.
  c) False. There is a 1-in-20 chance.
  d) True.
  e) False. $P < 0.05$ gives this level of significance.

60. a) True.
  b) True.
  c) True.
  d) True.
  e) False.

Exam no. 3   Questions

1. **Concerning biological electrical potentials:**
   a) EEG signals have an amplitude of up to 100 mV.
   b) Surface electrodes used for recordings should have an impedance >50 kOhm.
   c) The silver/silver chloride electrode is used to detect surface potentials because it has a very low resistance.
   d) EMG potentials tend to have a higher amplitude and shorter duration than ECG potentials.
   e) Evoked potentials are the electrophysiological response of the nervous system to stimulation.

2. **Concerning osmosis:**
   a) It is the movement of solute across a semi-permeable membrane.
   b) It generates a pressure which is expressed as osmolarity.
   c) 1 osmole of a substance is its molecular weight in g.
   d) The osmotic pressure is 22.4 atmospheres when 1 osmole of a substance is dissolved in 1 l of water.
   e) Osmolarity may be measured using the principle of freezing point depression.

3. **The following statements are true:**
   a) Henry's Law states that at constant temperature the volume of a fixed mass of gas is inversely proportional to its pressure.
   b) Dalton's Law states that at constant pressure the volume of a fixed mass of gas is proportional to its absolute temperature.
   c) Avogadro's hypothesis states that equal volumes of gases at the same temperature and pressure contain the same number of molecules.
   d) 1 mole of gas occupies 22.4 l at 0°C and 760 mmHg pressure.
   e) 1 mole of a gas at 0°C and 760 mmHg contains 6.02×10^{23} molecules.

4. Regarding capnography:
a) End-tidal CO_2 equals the arterial CO_2 tension.
b) The wavelength of light used is 940 nm.
c) In a side stream analyser the transit time of a sample from the breathing circuit to the analyser is between 5 and 10 s.
d) The rise time of a capnometer is the time taken for the analyser to register a change from 10 to 90% of the final value.
e) When used with closed systems, provision must be made to return the sampled gas to the breathing circuit.

5. The following measurements may be performed using a pulmonary artery catheter:
a) Left ventricular end-diastolic pressure.
b) Cardiac output.
c) Mixed venous oxygen saturation.
d) Right ventricular ejection fraction.
e) Central venous pressure.

6. In a normal recording of a 12-lead ECG:
a) The frontal axis lies between 0 and 90°.
b) The PR interval should be <0.12 ms.
c) T waves represent atrial repolarization.
d) The QRS complex coincides with ventricular ejection.
e) The T waves occur during ventricular systole.

7. When an automatic oscillometric blood pressure monitor is used:
a) The most accurate pressure displayed is the mean arterial pressure.
b) Compared with direct pressure measurements, it tends to over-read at high blood pressures.
c) At pressures of <80 mmHg, it tends to over-read compared with direct measurements.
d) Maximum arterial pulsations are detected at diastolic pressure.
e) A cuff which is too small will lead to over-estimation of the blood pressure.

8. The adrenal medulla:
a) Secretes adrenaline, noradrenaline and dopamine.
b) Is innervated by postganglionic sympathetic neurons.
c) Secretes steroid hormones in small amounts.
d) Is affected by ACTH, secreted by the anterior pituitary.
e) Is usually hypertrophied in acromegaly.

9. Na^+/K^+-ATPase:
a) Catalyses the formation of ATP from ADP.
b) Transports Na^+ ions out of cells.
c) Transports K^+ ions out of cells.
d) Is inhibited by ouabain.
e) Is an electrogenic pump.

10. Erythropoietin:
a) Is a circulating glycoprotein.
b) Secretion is stimulated by hypoxia.
c) Secretion is inhibited at high altitudes.
d) Is synthesized in the kidneys and liver.
e) Diverts stem cells from the leukocyte line to the erythrocyte line.

11. Bronchial smooth muscle:
a) Constricts in response to atropine and histamine.
b) Is relaxed by sympathomimetic agents.
c) Is relaxed by inhaled steroids.
d) Has a circadian rhythm with maximal dilatation in the early hours.
e) Is constricted by leukotrienes.

12. A substance used to measure glomerular filtration rate should:
a) Be secreted by the renal tubules.
b) Be highly protein bound.
c) Not be metabolized in the kidneys.
d) Be chemically inert.
e) Be an osmotic diuretic.

13. **The following events occur in a healthy individual during acclimatization to an altitude of 3500 m (10 800 ft):**
    a) An increase in red cell 2,3-DPG.
    b) A reduction in erythropoietin secretion.
    c) A fall in the myoglobin content of myocytes.
    d) Hyperventilation.
    e) Development of a metabolic alkalosis.

14. **During the cardiac cycle:**
    a) Tachycardia shortens the duration of diastole more than systole.
    b) At the end of systole the left ventricle is empty of blood.
    c) The mitral and tricuspid valves close simultaneously.
    d) Atrial contraction occurs at the start of diastole.
    e) The pulmonary valve closes before the aortic valve.

15. **Insulin:**
    a) Is an anabolic hormone.
    b) Promotes glycogenolysis.
    c) Is required for glucose uptake by brain and kidneys.
    d) Promotes gluconeogenesis.
    e) Stimulates the Na^+/K^+-ATPase pump.

16. **Immunoglobulins:**
    a) Bind to and neutralize some protein toxins.
    b) Block the attachment of viruses to cells.
    c) Opsonize bacteria.
    d) Activate complement.
    e) Activate natural killer cells.

17. **Bile acids:**
    a) Are based on the same molecular structure as cholesterol, vitamin D and steroids.
    b) Cause jaundice when secreted in excess.
    c) Play a role in the emulsification of fat prior to digestion.
    d) Undergo insignificant enterohepatic circulation.
    e) Are essential for adequate haemostatic activity.

18. An infusion of dopamine at 4 µg/kg/h:
a) Increases cardiac output.
b) Produces a diuresis.
c) Increases the systemic vascular resistance.
d) Increases the pulmonary vascular resistance.
e) Is a respiratory stimulant.

19. Fentanyl citrate:
a) May be absorbed transdermally.
b) Undergoes enterohepatic recirculation.
c) Is contraindicated for epidural or subarachnoid injection.
d) Has a pK_a of 8.4.
e) In a dose of 1–2 µg/kg obtunds the pressor response to laryngoscopy and intubation.

20. Adenosine:
a) Is formed by dephosphorylation of the adenine nucleotides ATP, ADP and AMP.
b) Should be administered into a central vein.
c) Is metabolized and excreted by the kidneys.
d) Potentiates the stimulating effects of catecholamines on the myocardium.
e) Commonly produces the side effects of dyspnoea and facial flushing.

21. In a patient taking warfarin:
a) Over 98% of circulating warfarin is protein bound and inactive.
b) Concurrent use of aspirin will produce a fall in the INR.
c) Chronic alcohol ingestion will raise the INR.
d) Vitamin K supplements are advisable.
e) Cimetidine enhances the anticoagulant effect.

22. Vecuronium:
a) Is a biquaternary aminosteroid.
b) Is stable in solution.
c) Causes systemic histamine release.
d) Is mainly excreted in bile.
e) Often causes a troublesome bradycardia.

23. First-order kinetics:
   a) Causes elimination of drugs at a uniform rate.
   b) Produce a straight line if drug concentration is plotted against time.
   c) May become saturated and display zero-order behaviour.
   d) Do not apply to phenytoin.
   e) Apply only to drugs which are protein bound.

24. A dose of 600–900 mg/day aspirin (acetylsalicylic acid):
   a) Is antipyretic.
   b) Reduces the bleeding time.
   c) Inhibits the enzyme cyclooxygenase.
   d) May cause a metabolic acidosis.
   e) May cause a normochromic normocytic anaemia.

25. When using a laryngeal mask airway in children:
   a) The size 2 mask requires 20 ml of air to inflate the cuff.
   b) The size 2½ mask is recommended for use in children weighing between 20 and 30 kg.
   c) It is not suitable for use in children aged <1 year.
   d) A size 1 mask requires 6 ml of air to inflate the cuff.
   e) The reinforced mask should always be used.

26. The following drugs are known to cause cholestatic jaundice:
   a) Halothane.
   b) Erythromycin.
   c) Amiodarone.
   d) Diclofenac.
   e) Diazepam.

27. Hepatic blood flow is decreased by:
   a) Halothane.
   b) Cimetidine.
   c) Somatostatin.
   d) Vasopressin.
   e) Propranolol.

28. Hepatic blood flow is the major determinant of the clearance of:
a) Warfarin.
b) Morphine.
c) Phenobarbitone.
d) Verapamil.
e) Isosorbide dinitrate.

29. The following are causes of a microcytic anaemia:
a) Vitamin B_{12} deficiency.
b) Sickle cell disease.
c) Renal failure.
d) Coeliac disease.
e) Iron deficiency.

30. In rheumatoid disease:
a) There is often a restrictive ventilatory defect.
b) Renal failure is a feature.
c) The disease causes a hypochromic anaemia.
d) Pericarditis is common.
e) If endotracheal intubation is indicated, it must be performed fibreoptically.

31. Diazepam:
a) Acts centrally to inhibit release of the neurotransmitter gamma amino-butyric acid.
b) Has no active metabolites.
c) Is water soluble.
d) Should not be used in children <3 years old.
e) Has a reduced duration of action in patients taking cimetidine because of hepatic enzyme induction.

32. Subarachnoid anaesthesia:
a) Must be performed at the same dermatomal level as the surgical procedure.
b) Is contraindicated in patients taking aspirin.
c) Is ideal for day case surgery.
d) Must be preceded by a preload of 1500 ml crystalloid.
e) May reduce the incidence of deep vein thrombosis.

33. Features of dystrophica myotonica include:
a) Autosomal dominant inheritance.
b) Cataracts.
c) Impaired neuromuscular conduction.
d) Hypertension.
e) Cardiomyopathy.

34. The following are true of halothane:
a) MAC is 1.15%.
b) It does not cause potentiation of neuromuscular blockade.
c) The saturated vapour pressure at 20°C is 243 mmHg.
d) Roughly 98% of inspired halothane is exhaled.
e) It is not influenced by the second gas effect.

35. Nitric oxide (NO):
a) Is the active ingredient of glyceryl trinitrate.
b) Is administered intravenously.
c) Is usually administered in doses of 10–50 ppm.
d) Concentrations can be measured by electrochemoluminescence.
e) Concentrations may be measured by telephotometry.

36. Compared with the non-pregnant state, changes which are seen in the third trimester include:
a) An increase in minute volume.
b) An increase in functional residual capacity (FRC).
c) An increase in respiratory rate.
d) An increase in tidal volume.
e) A decrease in oxygen consumption.

37. In a 3-year-old boy (15 kg) who has undergone nephrectomy, appropriate doses of analgesic drugs are:
a) Intravenous infusion of morphine sulphate 10–40 μg/kg/h.
b) Morphine sulphate 5 mg IM 3-hourly.
c) Paracetamol 120 mg 4-hourly.
d) Aspirin 300 mg.
e) Diamorphine 1–1.5 mg IM 3-hourly.

38. Causes of atrial fibrillation include:
a) Alcohol.
b) Hypoxia.
c) Hypokalaemia.
d) Pulmonary embolus.
e) Pneumonectomy.

39. Features associated with Fallot's tetralogy include:
a) Pulmonary stenosis.
b) Atrial septal defect.
c) Ventricular septal defect (VSD).
d) Apnoeic attacks.
e) Left ventricular hypertrophy.

40. Ropivacaine:
a) Is produced as a pure form of the 'S' enantiomer.
b) Is more lipid soluble than bupivacaine.
c) Has a higher plasma clearance than bupivacaine.
d) Is less cardiotoxic than lignocaine.
e) Produces a motor block which is slower in onset, less intense and of shorter duration than that seen after an equivalent dose of bupivacaine.

41. The following are contraindications to day case anaesthesia and surgery:
a) Age >70 years.
b) Non-insulin-dependent diabetes mellitus.
c) The patient lives alone.
d) Anticipated requirement for endotracheal intubation during anaesthesia.
e) The patient has no access to a telephone at home.

42. In non-insulin-dependent diabetes:
a) Gluconeogenesis is increased.
b) Insulin secretion is usually impaired.
c) There is usually microalbuminuria.
d) Treatment with insulin is not required.
e) Hyperosmolar non-ketotic coma may be precipitated by sulphonylureas.

43. Hypercalcaemia causes:
a) Tetany.
b) Constipation.
c) Carpopedal spasm.
d) Renal calculi.
e) Hypoglycaemia.

44. In Cushing's syndrome:
a) 30–50% of sufferers are diabetic.
b) Total body potassium is reduced.
c) Plasma potassium is usually normal.
d) Metyrapone, an 11β-hydroxylase inhibitor, decreases cortisol production.
e) Patients show a fall in plasma cortisol at night.

45. In hyperthyroidism:
a) Thyroid stimulating hormone levels are low in Graves disease.
b) Neonates born to mothers with Graves disease do not become hyperthyroid.
c) Patients prefer warm environments.
d) Beta blockers reduce the production of thyroxine by the thyroid gland.
e) The clearance of propranolol is higher than normal.

46. Pre-renal renal failure is characterized by:
a) Urinary osmolality > plasma osmolality.
b) Decreased urinary sodium.
c) Increased urine:plasma ratio for urea.
d) Proteinuria.
e) Decreased urine:plasma ratio for creatinine.

47. In von Willebrand's disease:
a) There is X-linked recessive inheritance.
b) Factor VIII levels are reduced.
c) Intravenous DDAVP raises the concentration of circulating factor VIII and von Willebrand's factor.
d) The bleeding time is prolonged.
e) Tests of the intrinsic pathway are prolonged.

48. In anaphylaxis:
   a) Histamine is a positive inotrope and chronotrope.
   b) Histamine decreases systemic vascular resistance.
   c) Tryptase levels decline after mast cell degranulation.
   d) Colloids should be avoided during resuscitation.
   e) Hydrocortisone should be the first drug given in order to give it time to work.

49. In the CO_2 electrode:
   a) There is a hydrogen ion sensitive glass electrode enclosed in a buffer solution and a CO_2 permeable membrane.
   b) Samples are always measured at 37°C.
   c) The pH increases by 0.01 for every 0.1 kPa rise in pCO_2.
   d) The buffer solution neutralizes pH to allow measurement of the pCO_2.
   e) The response time is <5 s.

50. In an exponential function where t = time and K = the rate constant:
   a) The 'break away' or 'tearaway' function is defined by the equation $y = e^{Kt}$.
   b) The wash-out curve is defined by the equation $y = e^{-Kt}$.
   c) The wash-in curve is defined by the equation $y = 1 - e^{Kt}$.
   d) The wash-out curve is defined by the equation $y = e^{Kt}$.
   e) The wash-in curve is defined by the equation $y = 1 - e^{-Kt}$.

51. When measuring evoked potentials:
   a) An external stimulus produces an EEG response.
   b) Volatile anaesthetic agents increase the latency of brainstem waves.
   c) Changes in auditory evoked responses are independent of anaesthetic drug doses.
   d) Auditory evoked potentials give an indication of depth of anaesthesia.
   e) Somatosensory evoked potentials can be measured from a peripheral nerve.

52. Concerning humidity:
a) The absolute humidity is the number of grams of water vapour present per cubic metre of gas.
b) Relative humidity is the percentage saturation of air with water vapour at a given temperature and pressure.
c) Air which is fully saturated at 20°C remains fully saturated when warmed to 37°C.
d) Absolute humidity may exceed the value for saturated air at that temperature.
e) An increase in humidity increases the risk of static electricity sparks.

53. Carcinoid tumours:
a) Originate from goblet cells of the intestinal mucosa.
b) Produce the carcinoid syndrome in 75% of cases.
c) When they cause the carcinoid syndrome produce symptoms which are predominantly due to the release of large amounts of histamine.
d) May be treated preoperatively by octreotide.
e) Can result in fibrosis of cardiac valves.

54. An electric current at 50 Hz passing through the body via a skin contact:
a) Can be felt at 1 μA.
b) Causes pain at 5 μA.
c) Causes respiratory muscle spasm at 50 mA.
d) Causes ventricular fibrillation at 100 mA.
e) May pass safely through the myocardium if the maximum current is 100 μA.

55. Plasma cholinesterase:
a) Has a normal plasma concentration of 5–10 units/ml.
b) Is a lipoprotein synthesized in the liver.
c) Is found in erythrocytes and plasma.
d) When deficient prolongs the dibucaine number to around 60% in heterozygotes and around 80% in homozygotes.
e) Hydrolyses the amide type local anaesthetics.

56. In methaemoglobinaemia:
a) The iron in haem groups is oxidized from the ferric to the ferrous form.
b) Methaemoglobin normally makes up 1% of haemoglobin.
c) Symptoms are seen when the percentage of methaemoglobin exceeds 20%.
d) Cyanosis occurs when there is 50 g/l of methaemoglobin.
e) At arterial oxygen saturations above 85% a pulse oximeter will read 85% but will give an accurate reading at saturations below this.

57. In hypothermia:
a) Plasma glucose and potassium increase as temperature falls.
b) A diuresis occurs.
c) Neonates tend to shiver at higher temperatures than older children and adults.
d) The rectal temperature is usually higher than other central measurements of temperature.
e) A sympathectomized limb will not vasoconstrict.

58. In the glass electrode:
a) There are two electrodes each kept at a constant potential.
b) There is approximately 60 mV produced per pH unit change at 37°C.
c) The response is to hydrogen ion activity rather than concentration.
d) The bridge between the sample and the electrode is soaked with sodium chloride.
e) The temperature of the electrode is adjusted to that of the patient and the sample before measurement.

59. The standard deviation:
a) Is the sum of the squared deviations from the mean divided by the number of observations.
b) Is the square of the variance.
c) Is the square root of the variance.
d) In a normal distribution 68% of values lie within 1 standard deviation above the mean.
e) In a normal distribution 95% of values lie within 1 standard deviation above the mean.

60. Statistical sensitivity:
   a) Indicates the ability of the test to give a positive result when the condition in question is present.
   b) When over 90%, means the test is always useful.
   c) Refers to the ability of the test to give a negative result when the condition in question is absent.
   d) When high indicates that the false negative rate is low.
   e) When over 90%, indicates that the test is clinically important.

Exam no. 3   Answers

1. a) False.
   b) False.
   c) False.
   d) True.
   e) True.

2. a) False. Solvent.
   b) True.   Osmotic pressures may be expressed as osmolarity
            (osmoles/l of solution) or osmolality (osmoles/kg of
            solution). For dilute solutions these are nearly identical.
   c) False. This is a mole of substance. One osmole is the
            molecular weight in grams divided by the number of
            freely moving particles each molecule produces when
            dissolved.
   d) True.
   e) True.   Dissolved solute tends to reduce the vapour pressure of
            a solute at steady temperature. Raoult's Law states that
            the depression or lowering of vapour pressure of a
            solvent is proportional to the molar concentration of
            the solute. One osmole/l of solute depresses the
            freezing point by 1.86°C and use of this fact is made
            in determining the osmolarity of a solution by the
            depression of freezing point.

3. a) False. This is Boyle's Law.
   b) False. This is Charles' Law. For ideal gases, Boyle's Law and Charles' Law can be combined as PV = nRT; where n is the number of moles present, R is the molar gas constant, P = pressure, V = volume and T = absolute temperature.
   c) True.
   d) True.
   e) True. This is the Avogadro Constant.

4. a) False. In health, there is usually a difference of 0.5 kPa between the two values. This difference may be much larger in the presence of various respiratory and cardiac disorders.
   b) False. 4.28 μm.
   c) False. <1 s.
   d) True. The transit time and the rise time are the components of the response time of a capnograph. This should be as short as possible to make it a real-time monitor.
   e) True. In a fully closed system, the volume of gas removed by a side stream analyser (150 ml/min) is significant and should either be returned to the circuit or compensated for with an increase in fresh gas flow.

5. a) False. The actual measurement made, the pulmonary artery occlusion (or wedge pressure), is an indirect estimate of left atrial pressure which in turn is an indirect estimate of left ventricular end-diastolic pressure.
   b) True.
   c) True.
   d) True.
   e) True.

6. a) False. −30 to +90°.
b) False. 0.2 ms.
c) False. Atrial repolarization occurs during the QRS complex and the signal is overwhelmed by this complex. T waves represent ventricular repolarization.
d) False. The QRS complex occurs during the phase of isovolumetric ventricular contraction before ventricular ejection starts.
e) True.

7. a) True.
b) False. These machines tend to under-read very high pressures and to over-read low pressures.
c) True. Maximum pulsations are detected at the mean pressure. Diastolic pressure is taken as the point when oscillations decrease suddenly. Difficulty in detecting this point means the diastolic is the least accurate of the pressures displayed.
d) False.
e) True. Just as with a sphygmomanometer.

8. a) True.
b) False. The adrenal medulla is a modified post-ganglionic sympathetic fibre and is innervated by pre-ganglionic fibres.
c) False.
d) False. Adrenal cortex.
e) False.

9. a) False. Catalyses the hydrolysis of ATP to ADP.
b) True.
c) False. K^+ is moved into cells.
d) True. And other cardiac glycosides.
e) True. Since three Na^+ ions are removed from a cell for each ATP molecule hydrolysed compared with two K^+ ions entering the cell the pump produces net movement of positive charge out of cells.

10. a) True.
   b) True.
   c) False. Stimulated, which is the mechanism for the development of polycythaemia in people acclimatized to altitude.
   d) True.
   e) False. Increases the number of erythropoietin-sensitive *committed* stem cells, which are then converted to red blood cells.

11. a) False. Acetylcholine is a bronchoconstrictor via muscarinic receptors and atropine prevents this and may cause bronchodilatation.
   b) True.
   c) False. These have a stabilizing effect on cells involved in the inflammatory reactions which contribute to asthma but do not produce bronchodilatation directly.
   d) False. Maximal constriction at this time.
   e) True.

12. a) False. Secretion by the renal tubules will produce concentrations in the urine which depend on something other than glomerular filtration rate.
   b) False.
   c) True.
   d) True.
   e) False.

13. a) True. This increases the P_{50} of haemoglobin for oxygen and tends to increase oxygen delivery to tissues.
   b) False. Polycythaemia occurs to increase tissue oxygen delivery.
   c) False. This is increased to improve oxygen uptake into respiring tissues.
   d) False. Hyperventilation occurs in response to hypoxia.
   e) False. There is an increase in urinary bicarbonate excretion and a mild metabolic acidosis occurs in response to the respiratory alkalosis.

14. a) True. The duration of systole is more fixed than that of diastole. At a heart rate of 65/min, systole has a duration of 0.25 s and diastole 0.55 s. At a heart rate of 200/min, systole is shortened to 0.15 s while diastole is 0.14 s. Since ventricular filling and left ventricular myocardial perfusion occur during diastole, rapid heart rates may impair cardiac performance.

b) False. There is an end-systolic ventricular volume. The ratio of this to end-diastolic volume gives the ejection fraction which is a useful index of myocardial performance.

c) True.

d) False. The atria contract towards the end of diastole and augment the passive ventricular filling which occurs during most of diastole. The importance of this effect on cardiac output becomes more important at high heart rates where the duration of diastole is reduced and so is the amount of passive ventricular filling.

e) False. In inspiration, the aortic valve closes slightly earlier than the pulmonary valve, although this is not the case during expiration. This occurs because there is a reduction in the impedance of the pulmonary vascular tree during inspiration. The increase in venous return produces a longer period of right ventricular ejection and splitting of the second heart sound.

15. a) True. Anabolic in the sense that it promotes the uptake and storage of absorbed nutrients by tissues.

b) False. As part of its anabolic actions, insulin promotes the formation and storage of glycogen in liver and muscle.

c) False. These, along with red blood cells and intestinal mucosa, do not require insulin for glucose uptake.

d) False. Gluconeogenesis is the opposite of the actions promoted by insulin and involves catabolic activity as stores of glycogen, fat or protein are mobilized.

e) True. This is the basis of the hypokalaemic action of insulin.

16. a) True. Depending on the circumstances, immunoglobulins may perform all of these functions.
   b) True.
   c) True.
   d) True.
   e) True.

17. a) True. The cyclopentanoperhydrophenathrene nucleus.
   b) False. Bilirubin causes jaundice.
   c) True.
   d) False. In health, 90–95% of bile acids are absorbed from the small intestine and undergo enterohepatic circulation.
   e) True. They are required for adequate absorption of fats and the fat-soluble vitamins, including vitamin K.

18. a) True. Even 'renal dopamine' has an inotropic effect.
   b) True. Dopamine has a diuretic effect on renal tubules in addition to its vasodilator effects.
   c) False. This happens at higher infusion rates.
   d) False.
   e) False. Although dopamine is found in the carotid bodies, exogenous infusion does not stimulate ventilation.

19. a) True. Due to its high lipid solubility.
   b) True. This is not a clinically significant effect unless very high doses are used.
   c) False. Because of its lipophilicity, fentanyl is very useful for epidural and subarachnoid use.
   d) True.
   e) False. This requires a dose of 5–10 µg/kg.

20. a) True.
   b) True. Because of its very rapid elimination and transient effects, adenosine is often ineffective if administered peripherally.
   c) False. It is metabolized in erythrocytes and endothelial cells.
   d) False. Adenosine decreases the release of catecholamines from cardiac sympathetic fibres and attenuates their effects on myocardium.
   e) True. Common but transient side effects.

21. a) True.
 b) False. Salicylates have a high affinity for binding sites on albumin molecules and tend to displace warfarin molecules, causing an increase in the INR. The effect of this may be compounded by the separate anti-platelet effect of aspirin.
 c) False. Induction of liver enzymes by alcohol will increase the metabolism of alcohol and tend to reduce its effect.
 d) False. The pharmacological effect of warfarin depends on the inhibition of the action of vitamin K.
 e) True. Cimetidine retards oxidative hepatic drug metabolism by binding to cytochrome P450 and tends to enhance the effects of warfarin.

22. a) False. Vecuronium is a monoquaternary homologue of pancuronium and the molecules of both compounds are based on a steroid nucleus.
 b) False. In solution, vecuronium undergoes slow deacetylation at position three of the steroid nucleus. A solution will retain clinical activity for 24 h. To aid storage, the drug is supplied as a powder which must be dissolved before use.
 c) False. Compared with other relaxants (and like pancuronium) vecuronium does not cause clinically significant histamine release.
 d) True. This is the main route of excretion.
 e) False. Because of its lack of muscarinic activity, the heart rate may be relatively slow and any stimuli tending to cause a bradycardia will not be antagonized. Vecuronium has no intrinsic bradycardic activity.

23. a) False. This is the definition of zero-order kinetics. In first-order kinetics, the rate of elimination of a drug is proportional to its concentration.
 b) False. The plot of concentration against time will produce an exponential curve (the greater its concentration the faster a drug is metabolized). The semi-logarithmic plot of log. concentration against time is linear in this case.
 c) True.
 d) False. At low concentrations, phenytoin displays first-order kinetics but its elimination pathways are easily saturable and at therapeutic plasma concentrations it displays zero-order behaviour.
 e) False. Nonsense.

24. a) True. Its original indication.
  b) False. Because of its effects on platelets, aspirin increases the bleeding time.
  c) True. This is the basis of many of aspirin's therapeutic indications.
  d) False. This will not happen with therapeutic doses; only in overdosage.
  e) False. If aspirin causes gastrointestinal blood loss sufficient to cause anaemia, it will be microcytic and hypochromic.

25. a) False. 10 ml.
  b) True.
  c) False.
  d) True.
  e) False.

26. a) False. Halothane hepatitis is a form of hepatocellular jaundice.
  b) True.
  c) False. Rare episodes of liver toxicity are hepatocellular.
  d) False. Likewise.
  e) False.

27. a) True.
  b) True.
  c) True. Somatostatin, vasopressin and propranolol have all been used for the treatment of bleeding varices, since they tend to reduce portal venous pressure.
  d) True.
  e) True.

28. a) False.
  b) True.
  c) False.
  d) True.
  e) True.

29. a) False. A macrocytic anaemia.
    b) True.
    c) False. Usually a normocytic anaemia.
    d) True.
    e) True.

30. a) True.
    b) True.
    c) False. Rheumatoid disease causes a normochromic anaemia. A hypochromic picture may be superimposed on this because of blood loss caused by NSAIDs.
    d) False. Pericarditis is rare in rheumatoid disease and is usually asymptomatic.
    e) False. This may be indicated in some patients with an unstable cervical spine but is not usually essential.

31. a) False.
    b) False.
    c) False.
    d) False.
    e) False. Cimetidine inhibits hepatic cytochrome P450.

32. a) False.
    b) False.
    c) False.
    d) False.
    e) True.

33. a) True.
    b) True.
    c) False. The neuromuscular junction is normal. Dystrophica myotonica is an abnormality of calcium ion metabolism in muscle cells. The main problems from an anaesthetic point of view are the abnormal response to suxamethonium and anticholinesterases, along with respiratory muscle weakness and cardiac conduction abnormalities.
    d) False. Hypertension is not a specific feature of this condition.
    e) True.

34. a) False. This is the MAC of isoflurane; that of halothane is 0.75%.
   b) False. Halothane has a slight effect in potentiating the neuromuscular blockers. It is less than that of enflurane or isoflurane.
   c) True.
   d) False. 20% is metabolized.
   e) False.

35. a) True.
   b) False.
   c) True.
   d) True.
   e) False.

36. a) True. Up to 50% above normal. Arterial pCO_2 commonly falls to around 4 kPa.
   b) False. The FRC is decreased from 20 weeks and falls below closing volume in about half of women. This is one of the reasons why preoxygenation before a general anaesthetic is important because a low FRC means alveolar oxygen reserves are low.
   c) False. The increase in minute volume is due to an increased tidal volume rather than respiratory rate.
   d) True.
   e) False. Basal metabolic rate is increased because of the requirements of the fetus, uterus and placenta.

37. a) True.
   b) False. Too large a dose. It should be 150–200 µg/kg.
   c) False. Too small a dose. 15 mg/kg.
   d) False. Contraindicated in children <12 years old.
   e) True. 80–100 µg/kg.

38. a) True.
   b) True.
   c) True.
   d) True.
   e) True.

39. a) True. VSD, pulmonary stenosis, overriding aorta and right
ventricular hypertrophy.
  b) False.
  c) True.
  d) False. Cyanotic episodes or 'spells' may occur from 3 months
but are caused by spasm of the right ventricular
outflow tract.
  e) False.

40. a) True.
  b) False.
  c) True.
  d) False. Bupivacaine.
  e) True.

41. a) False.
  b) False.
  c) True.
  d) False.
  e) True.

42. a) True.
  b) True.
  c) True.
  d) False.
  e) False.

43. a) False. A feature of hypocalcaemia along with carpopedal
spasm.
  b) True.
  c) False.
  d) True.
  e) False.

44. a) True.
  b) True.
  c) True.
  d) True.
  e) False.

45. a) True.
    b) False.
    c) False. Patients are heat intolerant.
    d) False.
    e) True.

46. a) True.
    b) True.
    c) True.
    d) False.
    e) False.

47. a) False. Usually autosomal dominant.
    b) True. von Willebrand's factor protects factor VIII from breakdown.
    c) True.
    d) True.
    e) False. Usually normal in the autosomal dominant form.

48. a) True.
    b) True.
    c) False.
    d) False.
    e) False.
    British Journal of Anaesthesia (1995) **74**: 217–228.

49. a) False. The electrode consists of hydrogen ion sensitive glass.
    b) True. Irrespective of body temperature, samples are warmed to 37°C prior to measurement. A correction factor is required to obtain the true pH and pCO_2 if the body temperature is significantly different from this.
    c) False. Decreases.
    d) False. The buffer solution dissolves CO_2 and releases hydrogen ions which are measured by the electrode to give an indication of the pCO_2.
    e) False. Two or three minutes: CO_2 must diffuse across the membrane covering the electrode before reacting with the buffer and releasing hydrogen ions.

50. a) True.
  b) True.
  c) False.
  d) False.
  e) True.

51. a) True.
  b) True.
  c) False.
  d) True. This appears to be a promising method of producing a formal measurement of depth of anaesthesia but remains a research tool at present.
  e) True.

52. a) True.
  b) True.
  c) False.
  d) True. If water droplets are present in the air.
  e) False. Reduced.

53. a) False. Argentaffin cells of the small bowel.
  b) False. 5–25%.
  c) False. 5-HT (serotonin).
  d) True. This is a somatostatin analogue.
  e) True. Predominantly the right sided valves, producing pulmonary stenosis and tricuspid regurgitation.

54. a) False. 1 mA.
  b) False. 5 mA.
  c) True.
  d) True.
  e) False. 10 µA.

55. a) False. 80 units/ml.
  b) True.
  c) False. Not in erythrocytes.
  d) False. The normal genotype is 75–85%, heterozygotes 65% and homozygotes 20%.
  e) False. Ester type.

56. a) False. From ferrous to ferric.
    b) True.
    c) True.
    d) False. 15 g/l.
    e) False. The oximeter also tends to read 85% when the SpO_2 is lower than this.

57. a) True.
    b) True.
    c) False. They do not shiver.
    d) True.
    e) False. A direct response to cold.

58. a) True.
    b) True.
    c) True.
    d) False. Potassium chloride.
    e) False. The sample is measured at 37°C.
              Sykes, Vickers and Hull, *Principles of Measurement and Monitoring in Anaesthesia and Intensive Care*, (1991) third edition. Blackwell Scientific Publications.

59. a) False.
    b) False.
    c) True.
    d) False. Either side of the mean.
    e) False. Either side of the mean.

60. a) True.
    b) False.
    c) False.
    d) True. 1 – sensitivity = false negative rate.
    e) False.

Exam no. 4   Questions

1. The critical temperature of a gas is:
a) The temperature at which the gas liquefies at 1 atmosphere pressure.
b) 36.5°C for nitrous oxide.
c) The temperature above which the gas cannot be liquefied.
d) The temperature at which cylinders of the gas should be stored.
e) The temperature below which mixtures of gases may separate into the constituent gases.

2. In an exponential process:
a) The rate of change of a quantity at any time is inversely proportional to the quantity remaining at that time.
b) The process is theoretically of infinite duration.
c) The half-life is half the time taken for the process to be complete.
d) The time constant is the duration of the process had the original rate of change continued.
e) The rate constant is the reciprocal of the time constant.

3. Concerning radioactivity:
a) An alpha particle is a proton.
b) A beta particle is an electron.
c) A gamma ray is an electromagnetic wave.
d) The SI unit of radioactivity is the Curie.
e) Radioactive decay is a linear process.

4. Surface tension:
   a) Is expressed in Newtons/m.
   b) Is defined by the equation: 'pressure gradient across the walls of a tube = radius/tension'.
   c) Is the cause of the meniscus on a column of fluid.
   d) Is twice as high in a tube as in a sphere of the same radius.
   e) Is reduced in alveoli by the presence of surfactant.

5. In a normal capnogram trace:
   a) Inspiration is represented by the trace at or near baseline.
   b) In health, the sharp upstroke of the trace should be vertical.
   c) The plateau of the trace is due to alveolar gas.
   d) The end tidal CO_2 is very close to the alveolar pCO_2.
   e) The downstroke is caused by the inspiratory pause.

6. The brachial plexus:
   a) Includes the posterior primary rami of nerve roots C5 to T1.
   b) Passes between scalenus anterior and scalenus medius.
   c) Provides the nerve supply to the deltoid muscle.
   d) Carries no sympathetic nerve fibres.
   e) May be blocked by an injection of local anaesthetic in the axilla.

7. In the stomach:
   a) The parietal cells secrete hydrochloric acid and intrinsic factor.
   b) Mucus secretion is inhibited by prostaglandins.
   c) Acid secretion is stimulated by histamine via H_1 receptors, acetylcholine and gastrin.
   d) Emptying is inhibited by intraluminal lipids.
   e) Omeprazole inhibits gastric acid secretion by the H^+/K^+-ATP pump of gastric parietal cells.

8. During sleep:
   a) Dreaming occurs during rapid eye movement (REM) sleep.
   b) REM sleep occupies about 25% of sleeping time in normal adults.
   c) Prolactin secretion is increased.
   d) There is an increase in skeletal muscle tone during REM sleep.
   e) The EEG is flat during periods of non-rapid eye movement sleep.

9. Calcitonin:
   a) Is secreted by the parathyroid glands in response to a high ionized plasma calcium concentration.
   b) Acts on bone to reduce absorption.
   c) Decreases the amount of calcium excreted in the urine.
   d) Is a steroid hormone.
   e) When injected has a therapeutic role in Paget's disease.

10. Aldosterone:
   a) Is a mineralocorticoid hormone secreted by the adrenal medulla.
   b) Secretion is increased by a rise in plasma potassium concentration.
   c) Has a natriuretic effect.
   d) Secretion is increased in response to trauma and hypovolaemia.
   e) Is independent of the renin–angiotensin system.

11. When using capnography in an intubated patient:
   a) The $P_{ET}CO_2$ is an accurate indicator of P_aCO_2.
   b) The area under the curve represents tidal volume.
   c) Rebreathing is indicated by notches in the plateau of the trace.
   d) The peak value reached for end tidal CO_2 is equivalent to P_aCO_2.
   e) Inspiration is indicated by the abrupt fall in the end tidal CO_2 value at the end of the plateau.

12. A capnograph:
   a) Relies on the absorption of infra-red light of wavelength $43\,\mu m$.
   b) Is unaffected by the presence of anaesthetic gases.
   c) Requires a sample volume of 5–10 ml/min of gas.
   d) Should have a rise time of <400 ms.
   e) Depends on the fact that molecules with dissimilar atoms absorb infra-red light.

13. In normal cerebrospinal fluid:
a) There is a protein concentration of 0.5–1.0 mg/ml.
b) The glucose concentration is around 3 mmol/l.
c) The sodium concentration is around 4 mmol/l.
d) There are 4–6 × 10^9 white blood cells per mm^3.
e) The pressure is 6–15 cm H_2O.

14. Haemoglobin S:
a) Differs from haemoglobin A by a substitution of valine for glutamine on the alpha chains.
b) Is inherited as an autosomal recessive.
c) When present along with HbA as the sickle cell trait, confers resistance to falciparal malaria.
d) Is present in about 10% of people from affected ethnic groups.
e) Starts to precipitate or sickle at a pO_2 < 8 kPa.

15. The following inhibit platelet aggregation:
a) Heparin.
b) Thromboxane.
c) Bupivacaine.
d) Ca^{2+} ions.
e) Acetylsalicylic acid.

16. Myocardial perfusion:
a) Is 225–250 ml/min in adults at rest.
b) Increases as heart rate increases.
c) Occurs mostly during systole.
d) Is increased by adenosine and prostacyclin.
e) Is largely dependent on systolic blood pressure.

17. The following stimulate insulin secretion in normal individuals:
a) Hypokalaemia.
b) Glucagon.
c) Glucose.
d) Amino acids.
e) Catecholamines.

18. Cyclic AMP:
   a) Is formed from ADP by the enzyme adenyl cyclase.
   b) Is converted to 5'-AMP by the enzyme phosphodiesterase.
   c) Inhibits the enzyme protein kinase A.
   d) Is the intracellular second messenger for adrenaline.
   e) Is the intracellular second messenger for acetylcholine at nicotinic receptors.

19. 5-Hydroxytryptamine:
   a) Is found in the central nervous system, intestine and platelets.
   b) Is metabolized mainly to 5-hydroxyindoleacetic acid.
   c) May be antagonized by ondansetron and methysergide.
   d) Is a major inflammatory mediator in the periphery.
   e) Is involved in the central processing of nociceptive stimuli.

20. The following drugs may cause bronchoconstriction:
   a) Atenolol.
   b) Vecuronium.
   c) Morphine.
   d) Fentanyl.
   e) Atracurium.

21. The following drugs act by increasing intracellular cyclic AMP:
   a) Theophylline.
   b) Adrenaline.
   c) Enoximone.
   d) Sodium nitroprusside.
   e) Lorazepam.

22. Desflurane:
   a) Is a fluorinated methyl ether.
   b) Has an MAC of 6%.
   c) Should not be used with soda lime.
   d) Has a SVP at 20°C of 673 mmHg.
   e) Has a boiling point of 43°C.

23. Warfarin:
   a) Acts as a vitamin K substitute.
   b) Has an anticoagulant effect which may be monitored using the activated partial thromboplastin time.
   c) Is contraindicated during pregnancy.
   d) Acts as an antagonist to factors II, VII, IX and X.
   e) Has a half-life in the body of 2–3 h.

24. Desmopressin acetate (1-deamino-8-D-arginine vasopressin):
   a) Is an artificial analogue of antidiuretic hormone.
   b) May cause a form of diabetes insipidus when used therapeutically.
   c) Increases the plasma concentrations of factor VIII, von Willebrand's factor and tissue plasminogen activator.
   d) Has a therapeutic role in haemophilia and von Willebrand's disease.
   e) Can be used long term in haemophilia to reduce the requirements for blood products.

25. The effects of the following drugs are enhanced by the chronic ingestion of cimetidine:
   a) Warfarin.
   b) Theophylline.
   c) Phenytoin.
   d) Salbutamol.
   e) Aspirin.

26. The following features of a drug make it likely to be subject to important drug interactions:
   a) A steep dose–response curve.
   b) Protein binding.
   c) A narrow therapeutic range.
   d) If it inhibits the metabolism of other drugs.
   e) A prolonged elimination half-life.

27. The following drugs can cause hyperglycaemia:
a) Bendrofluazide.
b) Captopril.
c) Digoxin.
d) Beta blockers.
e) Hydrocortisone.

28. The following drugs impair the action of platelets:
a) Aspirin.
b) Warfarin.
c) Heparin.
d) Lignocaine.
e) Diclofenac.

29. Flumazenil:
a) Is a competitive reversible antagonist of benzodiazepines.
b) Increases the clearance of benzodiazepines.
c) Does not reverse the amnesia caused by benzodiazepines.
d) Has a terminal half-life of about 1 h.
e) After oral administration has a bioavailability of over 80%.

30. Hepatic blood flow is the major determinant of the clearance of:
a) Diazepam.
b) Phenytoin.
c) Lignocaine.
d) Propranolol.
e) Caffeine.

31. The application of 10 cmH$_2$O of positive end expiratory pressure (PEEP) without changing the F$_i$O$_2$ may cause:
a) An increase in arterial pO$_2$.
b) A fall in oxygen delivery to tissues.
c) A fall in CVP.
d) A rise in intracranial pressure.
e) Increased secretion of antidiuretic hormone.

32. Hyperkalaemia is associated with:
  a) U waves on the ECG.
  b) Tall peaked T waves.
  c) Absent P waves.
  d) Metabolic acidosis.
  e) Widening of the QRS complex on the ECG.

33. The following drugs are effective after transdermal absorption:
  a) Fentanyl.
  b) Hyoscine.
  c) Ibuprofen.
  d) Glyceryl trinitrate.
  e) Atropine.

34. The following may cause vasodilatation and hypotension:
  a) Phentolamine.
  b) Phenylephrine.
  c) Nifedipine.
  d) Morphine sulphate.
  e) Protamine.

35. Axillary brachial plexus block:
  a) Carries a significant risk of pneumothorax.
  b) Avoids the risk of intravascular injection.
  c) Reliably blocks the musculocutaneous nerve.
  d) Requires the injection of 20 ml of 0.75% bupivacaine.
  e) Does not reliably provide analgesia for a tourniquet.

36. The Mallampati classification of airways:
  a) Is performed with the patient supine.
  b) Requires the patient to phonate.
  c) Requires the head to be extended.
  d) Has a sensitivity in predicting difficulty in intubation of over 95%.
  e) Includes five grades of appearance.

37. The following are caused by chronic excess alcohol consumption:
a) Peripheral neuropathy.
b) Cardiomyopathy.
c) Osteoporosis.
d) Bronchial carcinoma.
e) Congenital fetal abnormalities.

38. Respiratory depression after the use of epidural opioids:
a) Always occurs within 6 h of administration.
b) Is more likely to occur with fentanyl than with morphine.
c) Is more likely if they are administered in the thoracic rather than the lumbar region.
d) Is prevented by the concurrent administration of other sedative drugs.
e) Does not occur when the technique is used for analgesia in labour because of maternal hyperventilation.

39. Morphine sulphate may be absorbed by the following routes:
a) Transdermal.
b) Subcutaneous.
c) Epidural.
d) Rectal.
e) Oral.

40. The pressor response to endotracheal intubation will be minimized by prior administration of:
a) Fentanyl 1 µg/kg.
b) Alfentanyl 1 µg/kg.
c) Clonidine 5 µg/kg as premedication.
d) Spraying the vocal cords with lignocaine.
e) Esmolol 2 mg/kg.

41. Cricoid pressure:
a) Is intended to prevent vomiting.
b) Should be applied firmly before the induction of anaesthesia.
c) Should be applied using two hands.
d) Is not necessary in elective cases.
e) Is intended to occlude the oesophagus.

42. The following devices will supply a fixed F_iO_2:
a) Hudson mask.
b) Nasal cannulae.
c) Venti mask.
d) Anaesthetic circuit.
e) Hyperbaric chamber.

43. Concerning methionine synthetase:
a) Nitrous oxide oxidizes the cobalt atom in methionine synthetase.
b) Methionine synthetase is inhibited by nitrous oxide.
c) Methionine synthetase is the enzyme which regenerates tetrahydrofolate from methyl-tetrahydrofolate.
d) Vitamin B_{12} is a cofactor of methionine synthetase.
e) Inhibition of methionine synthetase may lead to reduced synthesis of deoxythymidine and interfere with DNA synthesis.

44. Features of chronic renal failure include:
a) Osteomalacia.
b) Peripheral neuropathy.
c) Megaloblastic anaemia.
d) Raised alkaline phosphatase.
e) Hypocalcaemia.

45. When using a circle system with the vaporizer outside the circle:
a) A low resistance draw-over vaporizer should be used.
b) Inhaled concentrations of volatile agent approach those set on the vaporizer as fresh gas flow increases.
c) Hypoventilation reduces the inspired concentration of volatile agent.
d) An oxygen analyser is not required.
e) At fresh gas flows of <1 l, the inspired concentration of volatile agent may exceed that set on the vaporizer.

46. Rheumatoid arthritis is associated with:
a) A low ESR.
b) Thrombocytopenia.
c) Amyloidosis.
d) High plasma albumin.
e) Mitral stenosis.

47. Bronchiolitis:
a) Is caused by a pneumococcal infection.
b) Is commonest in children aged <1 year.
c) Causes obstruction to expiration with air trapping in peripheral airways.
d) Usually requires intubation with IPPV.
e) Usually lasts <72 h.

48. Concerning diabetes mellitus:
a) Poorly controlled insulin-dependent diabetics may have symptoms of hypoglycaemia at higher plasma glucose concentrations than well controlled patients.
b) Hyperosmolar non-ketotic coma is less dangerous than diabetic ketoacidosis.
c) Epidural analgesia reduces postoperative insulin resistance.
d) Autonomic neuropathy is more likely in poorly controlled than well controlled insulin-dependent diabetics.
e) Endotracheal intubation produces less of a pressor response in insulin-dependent diabetics than in non-diabetic patients.

49. The stress response to surgery includes:
a) Increases in ACTH, cortisol and growth hormone.
b) Increased lipolysis.
c) Protein catabolism.
d) Increased glucagon secretion.
e) Reduced insulin secretion.

50. Addison's disease:
   a) Is a form of secondary hypoadrenalism.
   b) Can be caused by steroid therapy.
   c) Is characterized by high ACTH and low cortisol levels in plasma.
   d) May involve crises characterized by hyperkalaemia, hyponatraemia and elevated urea.
   e) Requires a dose of maintenance cortisol of approximately 30 mg/day.

51. The treatment of bupivacaine induced cardiac arrest is likely to require:
   a) Rapid reversal of hypoxia and metabolic acidosis.
   b) Prolonged cardiopulmonary resuscitation.
   c) Lignocaine for the treatment of ventricular tachycardia.
   d) Control of convulsions to decrease hypoxia and lactic acidosis.
   e) Bretylium for the treatment of cardiac arrhythmias.

52. The intra-tracheal route of administration is suitable for:
   a) Calcium.
   b) Adrenaline.
   c) Atropine.
   d) Bicarbonate.
   e) Fluid replacement.

53. In porphyria:
   a) Drugs which trigger attacks are inducers of the cytochrome P450 system.
   b) Attacks may be triggered by barbiturates, cimetidine, metoclopramide and nitrazepam.
   c) Attacks may be triggered by adrenaline, tubocurarine, suxamethonium and bupivacaine.
   d) Regional anaesthesia is contraindicated.
   e) Attacks may be triggered by steroids.

54. Concerning liquid manometers:
   a) A mercury barometer has a vacuum above the mercury and measures absolute pressure.
   b) Gauge pressure is pressure in excess of atmospheric pressure.
   c) In a mercury sphygmomanometer the markings for mm of mercury are 1 mm apart.
   d) In a tube <1 cm diameter, surface tension causes a water meniscus to over-read and a mercury meniscus to under-read pressure.
   e) Gauge pressure is measured with an open-ended barometer.

55. The normal ejection fraction is:

   a) $\dfrac{\text{End-diastolic volume minus end-systolic volume}}{\text{end-systolic volume}}$.

   b) $\dfrac{\text{End-systolic volume minus end-diastolic volume}}{\text{end-diastolic volume}}$.

   c) $\dfrac{\text{End-diastolic volume minus end-systolic volume}}{\text{end-diastolic volume}}$.

   d) 60–70% in the left ventricle.
   e) 60–70% in the right ventricle.

56. Duchenne muscular dystrophy:
   a) Displays X-linked recessive inheritance.
   b) Affects all skeletal muscle except the diaphragm.
   c) Is a contraindication to the use of suxamethonium.
   d) Involves atrophy of the myocardium.
   e) Produces early cardiac problems and later respiratory problems.

57. In the treatment of self poisoning:
   a) Activated charcoal prevents absorption of drug.
   b) Repeated doses of activated charcoal enhance elimination of drugs even after drug absorption from the gut.
   c) Alcohol intoxication is complicated by hyperglycaemia.
   d) N-Acetylcysteine is contraindicated in asthmatics.
   e) N-Acetylcysteine may cause hypotension and platelet dysfunction.

58. Methaemoglobinaemia may be caused by:
a) Aniline dyes.
b) Prilocaine.
c) EMLA cream.
d) Nitrates.
e) Methylene blue.

59. When using electromyography:
a) The normal nerve conduction velocity is 40–70 m/s.
b) Median nerve conduction velocity is normal in syringomelia.
c) The technique can distinguish between nerve, motor end-plate and muscle disease.
d) Conduction distal to a neuropraxia is abnormal.
e) It can be used to assess the depth of anaesthesia.

60. The statistical specificity of a test:
a) Refers to the ability of a test to give a positive result when the condition of interest is present.
b) When over 90%, indicates that the test is always useful.
c) Refers to the ability of the test to give a negative result when the condition referred to is absent.
d) When high means the false positive rate is low.
e) When over 90%, indicates that the test is clinically important.

Exam no. 4   Answers

1. a) False. Critical temperature is defined as the temperature
above which a gas cannot be liquefied. For oxygen this
is −119°C and for nitrous oxide 36.5°C.
  b) True.
  c) True.
  d) False.
  e) False.

2. a) False. It is directly proportional and this is the definition of
an exponential process.
  b) True.   Mathematical analysis of an exponential function gives
an infinite duration. Clearly no biological process can
have an infinite duration.
  c) False. It is the time taken for the quantity in question to fall
to half its original value. This is one method of
quantifying the behaviour of an exponential function.
  d) True.   This and the rate constant are alternative ways of
quantifying the behaviour of an exponential function.
  e) True.

3. a) False. An alpha particle is a combination of two protons and
two neutrons, i.e. a helium-4 nucleus.
  b) True.
  c) True.
  d) False. This unit is obsolete. The SI unit is the Becquerel (Bq)
which equals one nuclear transformation per second.
  e) False. It is an exponential process where the rate of
radioactive decay at a given time will depend on the
amount of radioactivity present.

4. a) True.

b) False. For a cylinder Laplace's Law is pressure = tension/radius. As the pressure falls, if the tension across the walls is kept constant, the radius tends to fall and may lead to collapse of the tube (or sphere), as in bronchi and alveoli during expiration.

c) True.

d) False. In a sphere, the pressure generated by surface tension is double that generated by the same tension in a tube of the same radius because there are two planes of curvature:

$$\text{pressure gradient} = \frac{2 \times \text{tension}}{\text{radius}}.$$

e) True. Lack of surfactant in ARDS and premature neonates is a cause of alveolar collapse.

5. a) False. The trace at zero or baseline represents early expiration, when CO_2–free gas from the anatomical dead space is sampled. In the absence of rebreathing, this should produce a trace at zero on the monitor.

b) False. The upstroke is caused by alveolar gas beginning to be measured. This would be vertical if all alveoli emptied simultaneously with the same time constants. Even in health this is not the case and so the upstroke is slurred. This effect is more pronounced in respiratory disease.

c) True.

d) True.

e) False. The downstroke is caused by inspiration.

6. a) False.

b) True.

c) True.

d) False.

e) True.

7. a) True.
b) False.
c) False. H_2 receptors.
d) True.
e) True.

8. a) True.
b) True.
c) True.
d) False. A decrease.
e) False.

9. a) False. Calcitonin is secreted by the thyroid gland.
b) True.
c) False. Urinary calcium excretion is increased.
d) False. Calcitonin is a peptide.
e) True.

10. a) False. Adrenal cortex – zona fasciculata.
b) True. This is a very potent stimulus to aldosterone secretion.
c) False. Preserves circulating volume.
d) True. Angiotensin II is a stimulus to aldosterone secretion.
e) False.

11. a) False.
b) False.
c) False.
d) False.
e) True.

12. a) False.
b) False.
c) False.
d) True.
e) True.

13. a) False. The protein concentration is normally <0.4 mg/ml and values in excess of this indicate infection or inflammation.
b) True.
c) False.
d) False.
e) True. Strictly speaking, cm of CSF.

14. a) False. This substitution occurs in the beta chains.
  b) False. Autosomal co-dominant.
  c) True.
  d) True.
  e) False. HbS starts to sickle at <5.5 kPa in sickle cell anaemia and around 2.7 kPa in sickle cell trait.

15. a) False.
  b) False. A potent stimulator of platelet aggregation produced by platelets.
  c) True. A well described effect of local anaesthetics both *in vitro* and *in vivo*.
  d) False.
  e) True. This action is the basis of the protective effect of aspirin against vascular thrombosis.

16. a) True. Making allowances for individual variation, these are the values given most commonly in textbooks of physiology and, like the blood flow to the brain, liver and kidneys, should be memorized.
  b) False. Perfusion of the major muscle mass of the heart, the left ventricle, occurs during diastole and is decreased as heart rate increases; particularly at rates in excess of 100/min.
  c) False. Two-thirds of the perfusion of the left ventricular muscle occurs during diastole because the tension generated during systole prevents perfusion of the subendocardial myocardium; although perfusion of more superficial regions will still occur. Other areas of the myocardium, i.e. the right ventricle and atria, generate lower pressures during systole and will be perfused during this time.
  d) True. These are physiological vasodilators. They may not dilate vessels which are atheromatous.
  e) False. Diastolic pressure, or more accurately the difference between diastolic pressure and end-diastolic ventricular wall tension, is a crucial determinant of myocardial perfusion.

17. a) False. Hypokalaemia reduces insulin secretion and
hypokalaemic patients often have an impaired glucose
tolerance.
 b) True. Glucagon has a direct action on the pancreas and an
indirect action via its catabolic actions.
 c) True.
 d) True.
 e) False.

18. a) False. Formed from ATP.
 b) True.
 c) False. It activates this enzyme which catalyses the
phosphorylation of intracellular proteins and so
changes their conformation and alters their activity.
 d) True.
 e) False. Acetylcholine works by altering ion fluxes across cell
membranes at these receptors.

19. a) True.
 b) True.
 c) True.
 d) True.
 e) True.
British Journal of Anaesthesia (1994) **73**: 395–407.

20. a) True. A well recognized side effect of beta blockers.
 b) False. Vecuronium is not associated with histamine release.
 c) True. Morphine is usually safe in asthmatics but occasionally
causes bronchospasm due to histamine release.
Fentanyl is free of this effect.
 d) False.
 e) True. Atracurium often causes histamine release when
>0.5 mg/kg is injected quickly.

21. a) True.
   b) True.
   c) True.
   d) False.
   e) False.

22. a) True.
   b) True.
   c) False. Desflurane is very stable in soda lime and, because of its cost, will probably always be used in semi-closed systems.
   d) True.
   e) False. Desflurane is very volatile and boils at 23°C, which means that it requires a pressurized vaporizer.

23. a) False.
   b) False. This is the test used to monitor the effects of heparin. Warfarin treatment is assessed using the prothrombin time.
   c) True. Because of the high risks of fetal abnormalities and fetal bleeding, warfarin would only be given to a pregnant woman in the most unusual circumstances.
   d) False. It reduces the formation of these factors rather than competes with them.
   e) False. The $t_{1/2}$ for warfarin is 48–72 h.

24. a) True.
   b) False. Desmopressin is the treatment for diabetes insipidus.
   c) True. These factors are mobilized from peripheral endothelial sites.
   d) True. It is helpful in those with low levels of factors who are not expected to bleed significantly but is inadequate for patients with minimal or absent endogenous levels of factors, or for major trauma or surgery.
   e) False. There is a rapid development of tachyphylaxis to the coagulant effects of desmopressin (but not to the antidiuretic effects) because of depletion of peripheral stores of these factors.

25. a) True.   Cimetidine is a potent inhibitor of oxidative hepatic metabolism by binding to cytochrome P450. This inhibits the metabolism of many compounds and three clinically important ones are warfarin, phenytoin and aminophyllines. Aspirin and salbutamol are not affected.
   b) True.
   c) True.
   d) False.
   e) False.

26. a) True.   This implies that small changes in plasma concentration produce significant changes in therapeutic effect and is particularly important in interactions which cause decreased efficacy of the relevant drug.
   b) False. Protein binding is only of relevance if the compound is very highly protein bound (>90%). Unless a drug is highly protein bound, the amount displaced by another compound, which is usually of the order of a few per cent, will make little impact on the circulating unbound concentration. Furthermore, if the drug has a large volume of distribution, any increase in circulating unbound drug will be diminished by subsequent distribution.
   c) True.   Any increases in concentration are likely to produce adverse effects in this case.
   d) True.   Almost by definition this suggests that such a compound will be a potent cause of drug interactions.
   e) False. This is not particularly relevant.

27. a) True.   This is a recognized side effect of thiazide diuretics and beta blockers.
   b) False.
   c) False. Hyperglycaemia is not seen with digoxin or captopril.
   d) True.
   e) True.   A well known side effect of steroids.

28. a) True.
b) False.
c) False.
d) True.
e) True.

29. a) True.
b) False.
c) False.
d) True. Hence its relatively brief effective duration and the danger of recurrence of benzodiazepine-induced effects, especially after an overdose.
e) False. There is a significant first-pass effect and the oral bioavailability is <20%.

30. a) False.
b) False.
c) True.
d) True.
e) False.

31. a) True. By increasing FRC, PEEP increases gas exchange and usually raises the pO_2, particularly if the lung pathology causes a reduced compliance, of which ARDS is a good example.
b) True. By reducing venous return and cardiac output, PEEP may reduce oxygen delivery to the tissues and measurements of cardiac output and mixed venous oxygen saturation can be made to assess this effect.
c) False. The CVP rises because the mean intrathoracic pressure is increased.
d) True. Although this is true, in the management of head injuries the maintenance of oxygenation is essential and PEEP is often used despite the risk of an increase in ICP. Direct measurement of ICP is often used in the management of severe head injuries and enables the effect of PEEP on ICP to be quantified.
e) True.

32. a) False.
b) True.
c) True.
d) True.
e) True.

33. a) True.
b) True.
c) True.
d) True.
e) False.

34. a) True.
b) False.
c) True.
d) True.
e) True.

35. a) False.
b) False.
c) False.
d) False. Too small a volume.
e) True.

36. a) False. Sitting upright.
b) False. Phonation is not part of the test described by Mallampati.
c) False. It is performed with the head in a neutral position.
d) False. No predictive assessment of difficult intubation has this degree of sensitivity.
e) False. Mallampati originally described three grades of appearance of the mouth. A fourth was subsequently added by Samsoon and Young.
Canadian Journal of Anaesthesia (1985) **32**: 429–434.
Anaesthesia (1987) **42**: 487–490.

37. a) True.
b) True.
c) True.
d) False.
e) True. Most seriously, the fetal alcohol syndrome.

38. a) False. May be delayed for >12 h, particularly in the case of morphine.
b) False. Because it is one of the most water soluble opioids, morphine is not absorbed into the epidural fat or spinal cord to the same extent as more lipophilic compounds and tends to remain free in the CSF to circulate and move rostrally.
c) False.
d) False. This will potentiate the effects of opioids.
e) False.
British Journal of Anaesthesia (1982) **54**: 479–486.

39. a) False. Morphine is too hydrophilic for this. Fentanyl may be given by this route.
b) True.
c) True.
d) True. There is a significant first-pass effect with the rectal and oral routes.
e) True.

40. a) False. A larger dose in the region of 5 μg/kg is required.
b) False. 10 μg/kg.
c) True.
d) False. This will require laryngoscopy which is usually more stimulating than the actual intubation.
e) True. A short-acting beta blocker.

41. a) False. Regurgitation.
b) False. At the induction of anaesthesia. Cricoid pressure is unpleasant and may cause nausea and vomiting.
c) False. It can be applied using two hands but classically the assistant uses one hand and gives the laryngoscope and endotracheal tube to the anaesthetist with the other.
d) False. It will be necessary if the patient is at risk of regurgitation and aspiration of gastric contents, e.g. hiatus hernia.
e) True.

42. a) False.
b) False.
c) True.
d) True.
e) True.

43. a) False.
b) True.
c) True.
d) True.
e) True.

44. a) True.
b) True.
c) False. Normochromic anaemia.
d) True. Usually raised as a result of osteomalacia and hyperparathyroidism.
e) True.

45. a) False. A high resistance plenum vaporizer is required which can accurately deliver high concentrations of volatile agent at low fresh gas flows.
b) True. At fresh gas flows above 2 l/min, there is little difference between the vaporizer setting and the inspired concentration of volatile agent.
c) False.
d) False.
e) False. The inspired concentration of volatile agent from a vaporizer outside the circle will not increase above the setting on the vaporizer.

46. a) False. The ESR is usually high.
b) False. Anaemia.
c) True.
d) False. This is usually low because of chronic inflammation and catabolism.
e) False. A possible consequence of rheumatic fever.

47. a) False. Usually respiratory syncytial virus.
   b) True. Peak incidence in children aged 3–6 months.
   c) True.
   d) False. About 5% of cases need to be ventilated. Among these there is a high proportion of children with congenital heart disease and neonatal ITU graduates with residual pulmonary damage from respiratory distress syndrome.
   e) False. 7–10 days.

48. a) True. *NEJM* (1988) **318**: 1487–1492.
   b) False.
   c) True. *British Journal of Surgery* (1988) **75**: 557–562.
   d) True. *BMJ* (1990) **301**: 565–566.
   e) True. *Canadian Journal of Anaesthesia* (1991) **38**: 20–23.

49. a) True.
   b) False. Decreased lipolysis.
   c) True.
   d) True.
   e) True.

50. a) False. Primary hypoadrenalism.
   b) False. This may precipitate Addisonian crisis but patients are not left with the disease.
   c) True.
   d) True.
   e) True.

51. a) True.
   b) True.
   c) False.
   d) True.
   e) True.
   Anesthesia and Analgesia (1985) **64**: 911–916.

52. a) False.
   b) True.
   c) True.
   d) False.
   e) False.

53. a) True.
   b) True.
   c) False.
   d) False.
   e) True.

54. a) True.
   b) True.
   c) False.
   d) True.
   e) True.

55. a) False.
   b) False.
   c) True.
   d) True.
   e) False. 40%.

56. a) True.
   b) False.
   c) True. It may cause potassium release and dysrhythmias.
   d) False. Hypertrophy.
   e) True.

57. a) True.
   b) True.
   c) False.
   d) False.
   e) True.

58. a) True.
  b) True.
  c) True.
  d) True.
  e) True.

59. a) True.
  b) True.
  c) True.
  d) False.
  e) True.

60. a) False.
  b) False.
  c) True.
  d) True.   1 – specificity = false positive rate.
  e) False.

Exam no. 5 Questions

1. Concerning electricity:
a) 1 coulomb is the quantity of electricity which passes a point when a current of 1 ampere flows for 1 s.
b) 1 volt is the potential difference which produces a current of 1 ampere when the rate of energy dissipation is 1 W.
c) The energy produced by an alternating current is less than that produced by a direct current with the same maximum amplitude.
d) Impedance refers to a resistance whose magnitude varies with frequency.
e) The unit of electrical power is the joule.

2. In laminar flow:
a) The flow rate is inversely proportional to the perfusion pressure.
b) The flow rate is proportional to the fourth power of the radius.
c) Density is the physical property which influences flow rate of a substance.
d) Fluid moves with uniform velocity.
e) A Newtonian fluid is required for laminar flow to occur.

3. The following physical principles are used to measure temperature:
a) An increase in the electrical resistance of a metal with temperature.
b) A change in the electrical resistance of a thermistor as the temperature changes.
c) The Seebeck effect.
d) The difference in the coefficients of linear expansion of two metals.
e) The Coanda effect.

4. Concerning humidity:
a) The factor which determines the amount of water vapour which a given volume of air can contain is the temperature.
b) As the temperature rises the amount of water vapour which a given volume of air can contain falls.
c) The absolute humidity is the maximum amount of water vapour which a given volume of air can hold at a given temperature.
d) Relative humidity is the ratio of the mass of water vapour present in a given volume of air to the mass of water vapour required to saturate the same volume of air at the same temperature.
e) Relative humidity may be expressed as the ratio of actual vapour pressure of water present to the saturated vapour pressure which is obtained at the same temperature.

5. Causes of an increased arterial to end-tidal pCO_2 gradient include:
a) Hypoventilation.
b) Rebreathing.
c) Hypovolaemia.
d) Adult respiratory distress syndrome.
e) Malignant hyperthermia.

6. The laryngeal mask airway:
a) Should not be re-used.
b) Can be used to administer intermittent positive pressure ventilation.
c) Is contraindicated in children aged <2 years.
d) Requires 20 ml of air to inflate the cuff of a size 3 mask.
e) Can only be used if anaesthesia is induced with propofol.

7. Human milk:
a) Has a pH of 6.7–7.4.
b) Has an osmolality of 315–325 mosm/l.
c) Is not secreted until after parturition.
d) Secretion requires the actions of both prolactin and oxytocin.
e) Contains no fat.

8. The nicotinic acetylcholine receptor:
a) Comprises six protein subunits.
b) Is only found at the neuromuscular junction.
c) Has a very high affinity for alpha bungarotoxin.
d) When stimulated by acetylcholine, changes shape to permit efflux of potassium ions from the muscle.
e) Has different structures in fetal and mature muscle.

9. In the fetal circulation:
a) The foramen ovale directs oxygenated blood from the left atrium into the right atrium.
b) The ductus arteriosus directs blood from the pulmonary artery into the aorta.
c) Oxygenated blood leaving the placental circulation has an oxygen saturation of about 94%.
d) The pulmonary vascular resistance is high compared with the systemic vascular resistance.
e) The ductus arteriosus usually closes within 4 h of birth.

10. The Bohr effect:
a) Reduces the P_{50} of haemoglobin for oxygen.
b) Occurs in the lungs.
c) Tends to increase the delivery of oxygen to tissues.
d) Is due to the fact that deoxyhaemoglobin binds H^+ ions more avidly than oxyhaemoglobin.
e) May be prevented by increasing the F_iO_2.

11. When using capnography in an intubated patient, the following tend to increase the arterial to end-tidal carbon dioxide tension difference:
a) A large right to left shunt.
b) Significant hypovolaemia.
c) A large air embolus.
d) Intubation of the right main bronchus.
e) Adult respiratory distress syndrome.

12. Sickle cell trait:
a) Is diagnosed by the Sickledex test.
b) Usually presents with a hypochromic microcytic anaemia.
c) Is not associated with episodes of sickling.
d) Is inherited as a sex-linked recessive disorder.
e) Precludes the use of tourniquets for surgery or intravenous regional anaesthesia.

13. The functional residual capacity:
a) Is higher in the supine than the upright position.
b) Usually falls after the induction of general anaesthesia.
c) Is increased by atropine.
d) When lower than closing volume, is associated with a fall in the alveolar-to-arterial oxygen gradient.
e) Is increased by the use of PEEP.

14. The transmission of nociceptive stimuli:
a) Is by A-delta and C fibres.
b) Is via synapses in the substantia gelatinosa.
c) Is by the posterior columns.
d) Is entirely somatic.
e) May be prevented by local anaesthetics.

15. The following are true of peripheral nerve fibres:
a) Nerves to skeletal muscle are unmyelinated.
b) Pain is transmitted in A-delta and C fibres.
c) C fibres are myelinated fibres with a diameter of <1 μm and a conduction velocity of 0.5–2 m/s.
d) B fibres are myelinated autonomic fibres.
e) A fibres range in size from 2 to 20 μm in diameter.

16. Immunoglobulins:
a) Are found as five groups of proteins.
b) Comprise two polypeptide chains.
c) Contain two light polypeptide chains.
d) Bind antigen with the constant portions of the polypeptide chains.
e) May be secreted into the gastrointestinal and genitourinary tracts and the bronchial tree.

17. Clonidine:
a) Is an agonist at alpha$_1$ receptors.
b) Is a potent analgesic.
c) May be administered by the epidural or subarachnoid routes.
d) May be used for premedication.
e) When used to provide analgesia, is devoid of effects on respiration.

18. Soda lime:
a) Contains 90% sodium hydroxide and 5% calcium hydroxide.
b) Must be completely anhydrous or it will become ineffective.
c) Contains ethyl violet to act as an indicator of exhaustion.
d) Absorbs CO_2 in an exothermic reaction.
e) Should fill 75–80% of the canister to ensure adequate contact with expired gases and complete CO_2 absorption.

19. Nifedipine:
a) Causes atrioventricular conduction block.
b) Antagonizes the effects of neuromuscular blockers.
c) Potentiates the effects of volatile anaesthetic agents.
d) Should be stopped 2 weeks prior to elective surgery.
e) Is a potent anti-dysrhythmic drug.

20. Captopril:
a) Inhibits the secretion of renin.
b) Causes an accumulation of bradykinin.
c) Inhibits the secretion of aldosterone.
d) May cause a rash, fever and taste disturbance.
e) Is a prodrug and is metabolized to its active form after absorption.

21. Sevoflurane:
a) Has a MAC of 6%.
b) Is stable in soda lime.
c) Has a blood-gas solubility coefficient of 0.6%.
d) Is a methyl propyl ether.
e) Undergoes metabolism to produce significant amounts of fluoride ion.

22. Dopexamine:
a) Is a synthetic phosphodiesterase inhibitor.
b) In a dose of 1–4 µg/kg/min has an affinity for both alpha and beta catecholamine receptors.
c) Has an affinity for dopaminergic receptors.
d) Causes a reduction in the neuronal re-uptake of catecholamines.
e) Usually produces a rise in heart rate and stroke volume along with a fall in systemic vascular resistance.

23. Ketamine:
a) Is highly protein bound.
b) Is mostly excreted by the kidneys as glucuronides.
c) Causes histamine release and bronchoconstriction.
d) Is antalgesic.
e) Is used in a dose of 2 mg/kg intramuscularly to induce anaesthesia.

24. The following drugs cross the blood–brain barrier:
a) Hyoscine.
b) Morphine.
c) Glycopyrrolate.
d) Vecuronium.
e) Atenolol.

25. 2% glutaraldehyde:
a) Is subject to an occupational exposure limit of 2 ppm.
b) Is used to disinfect endoscopic equipment.
c) Is used at a temperature of 45–50°C.
d) May cause asthma, dermatitis, sore throats and headaches in people exposed to it.
e) Is inflammable and should not be used in the vicinity of electrical equipment.

26. Gilbert's syndrome:
a) Affects 2–5% of the population.
b) Produces a conjugated hyperbilirubinaemia.
c) Produces jaundice during intercurrent illness, fatigue and fasting.
d) Is associated with normal liver histology.
e) Is caused by a deficiency of cytochrome P450.

27. Neostigmine:
a) Is a quaternary ammonium compound.
b) Has an elimination half-life of 10–20 min.
c) Undergoes substantial renal excretion.
d) May intensify a depolarizing neuromuscular block.
e) Is not used in infants because of its muscarinic effects, particularly bradycardia.

28. Cytochrome P450:
a) Is the terminal oxidase in the hepatic mixed-function oxidase enzyme system.
b) Structurally is based on a haem molecule.
c) Is inhibited by halothane.
d) Is inhibited by allopurinol.
e) Is responsible for the glucuronidation of many drugs.

29. Unnoticed endobronchial intubation during anaesthesia is likely to cause:
a) Hypoxia.
b) Hypercarbia.
c) Bronchospasm.
d) Pneumothorax.
e) Collapse of the contralateral lung.

30. Caudal injection of bupivacaine:
a) Does not cause sympathetic blockade.
b) Is contraindicated in day case surgery.
c) When performed in adults does not cause motor weakness of the legs.
d) Is free from the risk of subarachnoid injection.
e) Is performed via the sacral intervertebral foramina.

31. **Suxamethonium:**
a) Action is prolonged by tetrahydroaminotacrine.
b) Raises intra-ocular pressure to between 30 and 50 mmHg.
c) Is contraindicated in patients with head injuries.
d) Should be preceded by atropine.
e) May be reversed by anticholinesterase type drugs.

32. **Relating to cylinder supplies of anaesthetic gases:**
a) The tare weight is the weight of a full cylinder.
b) The pressure gauge gives an indication of the amount of nitrous oxide remaining in a cylinder.
c) They are filled to a pressure of 137 atmospheres.
d) Cylinders are made from titanium to provide strength.
e) Are unnecessary if the hospital has a spare central cylinder bank.

33. **EMLA cream:**
a) Contains lignocaine mixed with bupivacaine.
b) Has a total concentration of local anaesthetic of 2.5%.
c) Requires 30 min to produce analgesia for venepuncture.
d) Initially produces vasoconstriction in the underlying skin.
e) Requires penetration of the stratum corneum by local anaesthetic to be effective.

34. **Features which are predictive of difficulty in endotracheal intubation include:**
a) Weight >110 kg.
b) Thyromental distance >7 cm.
c) Limited extension of the atlanto–occipital joint.
d) A beard.
e) Protruding upper teeth.

35. **In haemophilia A:**
a) There is autosomal dominant inheritance.
b) The bleeding time is normal.
c) The prothrombin time (INR) is prolonged.
d) The deficient factor is factor VIII.
e) Treatment is usually in the form of fresh frozen plasma.

36. Features of the adult respiratory distress syndrome (ARDS) include:
a) A high pulmonary capillary wedge pressure.
b) An increase in lung compliance.
c) An increase in pulmonary shunt fraction.
d) Pulmonary hypertension.
e) Pulmonary fibrosis.

37. The following are required for a diagnosis of pre-eclampsia:
a) Oedema.
b) Gestation >16 weeks.
c) Diastolic blood pressure >110 mm Hg.
d) Systolic blood pressure >140 mmHg.
e) Thrombocytopenia.

38. In non-insulin-dependent diabetes:
a) Gluconeogenesis is increased.
b) Insulin secretion is usually impaired.
c) There is usually microalbuminuria.
d) Treatment with insulin is not required.
e) Hyperosmolar non-ketotic coma may be precipitated by sulphonylureas.

39. The combined oral contraceptive pill is a recognized cause of:
a) Deep venous thrombosis.
b) Hypertension.
c) Depression.
d) Acne.
e) Bruising.

40. The following features are characteristic of acute intermittent porphyria:
a) Hypertension.
b) Abdominal pain.
c) Photosensitivity.
d) Peripheral neuropathy.
e) Hyperglycaemia.

41. Hypothyroid patients:
a) Take longer to emerge from anaesthesia than normal.
b) Have a need for larger than normal induction doses of anaesthetic agents.
c) May require a lower minute volume than normal to maintain normocarbia.
d) Have an increased sensitivity to muscle relaxants.
e) Often have an associated adrenocortical insufficiency.

42. In Conn's syndrome:
a) There is secondary hyperaldosteronism.
b) The condition presents with hyponatraemia and hypotension.
c) Low plasma and total body potassium is reflected by a low urinary potassium level.
d) Patients are sensitive to non-depolarizing muscle relaxants.
e) Plasma renin is elevated.

43. In myasthenia gravis:
a) Muscles fatigue with repetition of an action.
b) Circulating antibodies to the acetylcholine receptor are elevated in 90% of cases.
c) The clinical severity of the disease is correlated with the antibody titre.
d) Intravenous edrophonium can make the weakness more severe.
e) There are increased numbers of acetylcholine receptors on the post-junctional membrane.

44. Bupivacaine toxicity:
a) Is more likely to occur in a hypovolaemic patient than a normovolaemic patient of the same weight.
b) Is prevented in the presence of inhalational anaesthetic agents.
c) Is characterized by a smaller difference between the plasma concentrations required for CNS and cardiac effects than lignocaine.
d) Is more likely in pregnant than non-pregnant patients.
e) Can be prevented by a benzodiazepine premedication.

45. 1 pascal equals:
a) $1\,N\,m^{-2}$.
b) $1\,kg\,m\,s^{-2}$.
c) $7.6\,mmHg$.
d) $1\,J\,m^{-3}$.
e) $1\,kg\,m^{-1}\,s^{-2}$.

46. When electroencephalography is used during anaesthesia:
a) A transition from fast to slow waves is seen at induction.
b) Alpha waves are increased during general anaesthesia.
c) High dose barbiturates initially increase 'fast' activity before 'slow' activity.
d) Enflurane causes increased voltages and frequencies enhanced by hypercapnia and light anaesthesia.
e) In an awake patient the dominant frequency is about 10 Hz.

47. Down's syndrome is associated with:
a) Cervical spine instability.
b) Sleep apnoea.
c) Hypothyroidism.
d) Difficulty with endotracheal intubation.
e) A requirement for smaller diameter endotracheal tubes than the size calculated on the basis of age.

48. Serotonin:
a) Is synthesized from tryptophan via 5-hydroxyindole acetic acid.
b) Promotes platelet aggregation.
c) Is a vasoconstrictor.
d) Increases gastrointestinal motility.
e) Is a neurotransmitter.

49. Q waves on the ECG:
a) Are a characteristic feature of sub-endocardial infarction.
b) To be considered significant, should last for 40 ms and have an amplitude over 25% that of the accompanying R wave.
c) Do not develop in the presence of left bundle branch block.
d) Appear within 24 h of a myocardial infarction.
e) May not be pathological.

50. In aortic stenosis:
   a) The cross-sectional area of the aortic valve must be reduced to $3\,cm^2$ to produce symptoms.
   b) Left ventricular volume increases early in the disease.
   c) Decreasing afterload increases the ejection fraction.
   d) The absence of left ventricular hypertrophy on the ECG excludes significant stenosis.
   e) A systolic blood pressure >180 mmHg excludes significant disease.

51. The central anticholinergic syndrome:
   a) Is due to excessive central cholinergic activity.
   b) May occur after prolonged sedation.
   c) May be caused by atropine, hyoscine and phenothiazines.
   d) May be caused by benzodiazepines and opioids.
   e) Is rapidly reversed with neostigmine 2 mg intravenously.

52. Nitric oxide:
   a) Has been identified as a neurotransmitter.
   b) Acts as a physiological vasodilator.
   c) Has a half-life of 5 min.
   d) Has effects which are localized by haemoglobin.
   e) Is an effector in the immune system inhibiting ATP and DNA synthesis in bacteria.

53. Features of cocaine intoxication include:
   a) Acute rhabdomyolysis.
   b) Coronary vasoconstriction.
   c) Hypertension and bradycardia.
   d) Prevention of noradrenaline reuptake at sympathetic nerve endings.
   e) Enhanced toxicity in patients with plasma cholinesterase deficiency.

54. Features associated with a good prognosis in cardiac arrest include:
a) An initial rhythm which is ventricular fibrillation.
b) A witnessed arrest.
c) Short time to initiation of resuscitation.
d) Short time to defibrillation.
e) The use of bicarbonate.

	Condition present	Condition absent
Test positive	A	B
Test negative	C	D

In the table above

55. Specificity is calculated by:

a) $\dfrac{A}{A + C}$.

b) $\dfrac{D}{D + B}$.

c) $\dfrac{B}{A + B}$.

d) $\dfrac{C}{C + D}$.

e) $\dfrac{A}{B + D}$.

56. Sensitivity is calculated by:

a) $\dfrac{A}{A + C}$.

b) $\dfrac{D}{D + B}$.

c) $\dfrac{B}{A + B}$.

d) $\dfrac{C}{C + D}$.

e) $\dfrac{A}{B + D}$.

57. The fraction of false positives is given by:

a) $\dfrac{A}{A + C}$.

b) $\dfrac{D}{D + B}$.

c) $\dfrac{B}{A + B}$.

d) $\dfrac{C}{C + D}$.

e) $\dfrac{A}{B + D}$.

58. The fraction of false negatives is given by:

a) $\dfrac{A}{A + C}$.

b) $\dfrac{D}{D + B}$.

c) $\dfrac{B}{A + B}$.

d) $\dfrac{C}{C + D}$.

e) $\dfrac{A}{B + D}$.

59. The positive predictive value is:

a) $\dfrac{A}{A + B}$.

b) $\dfrac{D}{C + D}$.

c) $\dfrac{B}{A + B}$.

d) $\dfrac{A}{A + C}$.

e) $\dfrac{A}{B + D}$.

60. The negative predictive value is:

a) $\dfrac{A}{A + B}$

b) $\dfrac{D}{C + D}$

c) $\dfrac{C}{C + D}$

d) $\dfrac{D}{B + D}$

e) $\dfrac{A}{B + D}$

Exam no. 5   Answers

1. a) True.
   b) True.
   c) True.   A more accurate indicator of the energy produced by
            an alternating current is the root mean square of the
            current because, for alternating current, the maximum
            current is attained for only a small fraction of each
            cycle.
   d) True.
   e) False. The unit of electrical power is the Watt.

2. a) False. Laminar flow is described by the Hagen–Poiseulle
            equation:

$$\text{Flow rate} \propto \frac{(P_1 - P_2)\,\pi\,r^4}{8\,\eta\,l}$$

            where P_1 and P_2 are the pressures at each end of the
            tube, r is the radius, l is the length of the tube and η is
            the viscosity of the liquid.
   b) True.
   c) False. The relevant physical property is viscosity – that
            property of a fluid which causes it to resist flow.
   d) False. During laminar flow, molecules travel with the greatest
            velocity in the axial line while those in contact with
            the walls of the tube travel much more slowly. The
            velocity of flow in the axial stream may be twice the
            average linear velocity of flow.
   e) True.

3. a) True.
   b) True.
   c) True. This is the physical principle of the thermocouple where, at the junction of two metals, a voltage is produced. The magnitude of this voltage is dependent on the temperature at the junction. If a circuit is made incorporating this junction and a second junction, kept at a constant temperature (the reference junction), the first junction can be used as a temperature probe.
   d) True.
   e) False. A principle of fluid mechanics.

4. a) True.
   b) False. It increases.
   c) False. It is the actual mass of water present in a given volume of air.
   d) True.
   e) True.

5. a) False. The increase in end-tidal CO_2 reflects a genuine increase in arterial pCO_2.
   b) False. There is also a rise in arterial pCO_2 here.
   c) True. There is a fall in pulmonary perfusion and a rise in the degree of V/Q mismatch occurs.
   d) True. V/Q mismatch is increased.
   e) False. A genuine rise in arterial pCO_2.

6. a) False. Laryngeal masks can be used up to 40 times and should be autoclaved between patients.
   b) True. This is true, although most people feel that they should not normally be used to administer planned IPPV lasting for more than a few minutes because of the risk of gastric dilatation. They may be useful in the management of a difficult intubation in a paralysed patient when this is a relatively minor consideration.
   c) False.
   d) True.
   e) False. Insertion is often easier after propofol than other methods of induction but the crucial requirement is for an adequate depth of anaesthesia rather than for any particular way of producing this.

7. a) True.
   b) False. Osmolarity is similar to that of plasma, around 286 mosm/l.
   c) False. Small amounts are secreted from the 5th month of pregnancy onwards.
   d) True.
   e) False. Variable amounts of fat are secreted, depending on maternal diet, the duration of lactation and the frequency of breast feeding.

8. a) False. It comprises five subunits – two alpha, one beta, one delta and one epsilon.
   b) False. Also found in autonomic ganglia and all over denervated muscles.
   c) True.
   d) False. Sodium influx.
   e) True. In fetal myocytes, there is a gamma subunit rather than an epsilon subunit.

9. a) False. Oxygenated blood is directed from the right to the left atrium.
   b) True.
   c) False. The S_pO_2 is about 80%, which falls to about 65% when placental blood mixes with portal blood during return to the right side of the heart.
   d) True.
   e) False. Functional closure of the duct takes several days.

10. a) False.
   b) False. The Bohr effect occurs in respiring tissues and produces a small (1–2%) increase in the amount of oxygen released from oxyhaemoglobin due to the low tissue pO_2.
   c) True.
   d) True.
   e) False.

11. a) True.
   b) True.
   c) True.
   d) False.
   e) True.

12. a) False. The Sickledex test is a commercial macroscopic test for deoxygenated insoluble HbS. It does not distinguish between the trait and sickle cell anaemia, is unreliable in patients <2 years of age and is subject to false positives. Accurate diagnosis of sickle cell trait or any haemoglobinopathy requires haemoglobin electrophoresis.

b) False. This is characteristic of sickle cell anaemia. In the trait, the Hb concentration and blood film are usually normal.

c) False. Sickling will occur at a $pO_2 < 2.7$ kPa.

d) False. Autosomal.

e) False. This is a debatable point but many would feel that if the use of a tourniquet offered clear advantages to the patient then it should be used. There is no clinical evidence of harm being caused in sickle cell trait by the correct use of a tourniquet.

13. a) False.

b) True.

c) True. Due to the slight bronchodilatation produced by atropine.

d) False. There is an increase in this gradient, i.e. a fall in arterial pO_2.

e) True. This is the explanation for the beneficial effect on oxygenation produced by PEEP.

14. a) True. Pain transmission is by both 'fast' A-delta and 'slow' C fibres.

b) True. The substantia gelatinosa comprises Rexed's laminae II and III and is important for the central transmission of pain and its modification by descending fibres and analgesics.

c) False. Pain is transmitted centrally by the spinothalamic tracts.

d) False. Sympathetic fibres are important in pain transmission and play a large part in the generation of various chronic pain syndromes.

e) True. Local anaesthetics are the only class of analgesic drugs used clinically which abolish pain by preventing central transmission of nociceptive stimuli.

15. a) False. These fibres are myelinated to ensure rapid impulse
        conduction and rapid coordinated movements.
   b) True.
   c) False. C fibres are unmyelinated and have a slow conduction
        speed.
   d) True.
   e) True.

16. a) True.   Immunoglobulins G, A, M, D and E.
   b) False. Four chains – two heavy and two light.
   c) True.   Either two κ or two λ light chains are found in each
        immunoglobulin molecule.
   d) False. The variable portions of the chains which form the
        antibody binding sites (Fab portions).
   e) True.   IgA.

17. a) True   Although primarily an alpha$_2$ agonist, clonidine
        stimulates inhibitory post-synaptic alpha$_1$ receptors.
   b) False.
   c) True.   Although used in this way, clonidine is not licensed for
        this indication.
   d) True.
   e) False. At doses of 4 μg/kg and above, there is a reduced
        sensitivity to carbon dioxide and the carbon dioxide
        response curve is shifted to the right, i.e. there is
        respiratory depression.
        Anaesthesia (1991) **46**: 1003–1004.

18. a) False. 94% calcium hydroxide, 5% sodium hydroxide, 1%
        potassium hydroxide, silicates and indicators.
   b) False.
   c) False.
   d) True.
   e) True.

19. a) False.
   b) False.
   c) True.
   d) False.
   e) False.

20. a) False. ACE inhibitors reduce the formation of angiotensin II from angiotensin I.
    b) True. Bradykinin is degraded by angiotensin converting enzyme.
    c) True.
    d) True. These side effects occur in 5–10% of patients.
    e) False. This is the case with enalapril rather than captopril.

21. a) False. 2%.
    b) False. Degraded slightly by soda lime.
    c) True.
    d) True.
    e) True. 22 mmol/l after 60 min anaesthesia at 1 MAC.

22. a) False. Dopexamine is a synthetic catecholamine.
    b) False. At therapeutic doses, it has no affinity for alpha receptors.
    c) True. This is partly responsible for the increased splanchnic perfusion produced by dopexamine.
    d) True. This is partly responsible for the inotropic effects of dopexamine.
    e) True.

23. a) False. Ketamine is only 10–12% protein bound.
    b) True. After conjugation in the liver by demethylation and hydroxylation. Among the metabolites is an active compound called norketamine.
    c) False. Ketamine is a bronchodilator and many anaesthetists would use this to induce a patient *in extremis* with severe asthma.
    d) False. A potent analgesic in subanaesthetic doses of about 0.5 mg/kg.
    e) False. This is the intravenous dose. When used intramuscularly a dose of 8–10 mg/kg is required.

24. a) True.
    b) True.
    c) False. As a quaternary rather than tertiary nitrogen compound, such as atropine and hyoscine, glycopyrrolate does not cross the blood–brain barrier and does not have central effects when used with neostigmine for the reversal of neuromuscular blockade.
    d) False. As charged quaternary nitrogen compounds, muscle relaxants do not cross the blood–brain barrier.
    e) True.

25. a) False. There is no UK exposure limit. In the USA it is 0.2 ppm.
    b) True.
    c) False. Room temperature.
    d) True.
    e) False.

26. a) True. Usually an asymptomatic condition.
    b) False. Unconjugated.
    c) True.
    d) True.
    e) False. Glucuronyl transferase.

27. a) True. As are acetylcholine and neuromuscular blockers.
    b) False. 20–80 min in patients with normal renal function.
    c) True. 50%.
    d) True.
    e) False.

28. a) True.
    b) True.
    c) False.
    d) True.
    e) False. Oxidation.

29. a) True.
   b) False.
   c) True. This is a potent cause of bronchospasm.
   d) False. Although a pneumothorax may occur because of the increased inflation pressure caused by bronchospasm and volume cycling without pressure limitation, it is unusual in this situation.
   e) True.

30. a) False.
   b) True. This is debatable but the incidence of motor weakness in the legs would make most anaesthetists avoid caudal blockade in day case surgery. However, it is commonly used in paediatric day case surgery.
   c) False.
   d) False.
   e) False. Sacral hiatus.

31. a) True.
   b) False.
   c) False.
   d) False.
   e) True. In phase II block.

32. a) False.
   b) False.
   c) False.
   d) False.
   e) False.

33. a) False. EMLA cream is a mixture of 2.5% lignocaine and 2.5% prilocaine, giving a total concentration of 5%.
   b) False.
   c) False. It requires application for an hour to exert a consistent effect.
   d) True. This is a minor drawback to its use. If applied for long enough the cream tends to produce vasodilatation.
   e) True. This is the main barrier to transdermal absorption of drugs.

34. a) True.   Several anatomical features have been shown to correlate in varying degrees with difficulty in endotracheal intubation. These include obesity (weight >110 kg), limited extension at the atlanto–occipital joint, protruding upper teeth and a thyromental distance of <6.5 cm. All of the methods used to predict difficulty in intubation suffer from limited sensitivity (false negatives) and specificity (false positives).

   b) False.
   c) True.
   d) False.
   e) True.

35. a) False.   X-linked recessive, which is why the majority of sufferers are male.

   b) True.   Platelet function is unaffected and so this test is normal.

   c) False.   The defect is in the intrinsic pathway, so the partial thromboplastin time is prolonged while the prothrombin time is normal.

   d) True.   This is the case in 95% of sufferers with haemophilia A. Those with haemophilia B are deficient in factor IX.

   e) False.   Treatment is usually with factor VIII concentrates.

36. a) False.   The PCWP should be low or normal in most cases. A high PCWP suggests that the oedema is cardiac in origin, although the two forms may occur in the same patient.

   b) False.   Pulmonary compliance is markedly reduced because of the inflammatory exudate in alveoli.

   c) True.
   d) True.
   e) True.   This is seen during the recovery phase of ARDS and is a common reason for prolonged respiratory impairment after resolution of the presenting illness.

37. a) False. The classification and definition of hypertensive disorders during pregnancy continue to be controversial. The International Society for the Study of Hypertension have produced definitions which are widely accepted. Oedema is not required for a definition of pre-eclampsia.
   b) False. 20 weeks.
   c) True. Greater than 100 mmHg on a single occasion or 90 mmHg on two or more occasions at least 4 h apart. The blood pressure must be measured correctly. Phase IV Korotkoff sounds are generally used in the UK and this is accepted by the ISSH.
   d) False. Systolic blood pressure does not appear in the definition.
   e) False. This is a complication of severe pre-eclampsia.
   British Journal of Anaesthesia (1996) **76**: 133–148.

38. a) True.
   b) True.
   c) True.
   d) False.
   e) False.

39. a) True. A rare but definite association, which is made more likely by the presence of other risk factors such as smoking, obesity and hypertension.
   b) True. This usually disappears when the oral contraceptive pill is withdrawn.
   c) True.
   d) True. Due to progestogens.
   e) False.

40. a) True.
   b) True.
   c) False. Not seen in the acute intermittent form of the disease.
   d) True.
   e) False.

41. a) False.
    b) False.
    c) True. Due to decreased metabolic rate.
    d) False.
    e) True.

42. a) False.
    b) False. Hypertension and a normal or high sodium.
    c) False. Elevated urinary potassium.
    d) True. Secondary to hypokalaemia.
    e) False. Decreased.

43. a) True.
    b) True.
    c) False.
    d) True. Indicative of cholinergic crisis due to excessive inhibition of anticholinesterase.
    e) False. Decreased.

44. a) True.
    b) False.
    c) True.
    d) True.
    e) False.

45. a) True.
    b) False. 1 Newton.
    c) False. 7.6 mmHg = 1 kPa.
    d) True. 1 Joule = 1 Nm.
    e) True.

46. a) True.
    b) False. These are seen in patients who are awake with their eyes closed.
    c) True.
    d) False. Hypocapnia and deep anaesthesia.
    e) True.

47. a) True.
   b) True.
   c) True.
   d) True.
   e) True.   *Paediatric Anaesthesia* (1995) **5**: 379–384.

48. a) False.   5-Hydroxyindole acetic acid is a breakdown product of serotonin.
   b) True.
   c) True.
   d) True.
   e) True.

49. a) False.
   b) True.
   c) True.
   d) True.
   e) True.

50. a) False.   This is the surface area of a normal valve.
   b) False.
   c) False.   The resistance to ejection is fixed.
   d) False.
   e) True.

51. a) False.
   b) True.
   c) True.
   d) True.
   e) False.   Physostigmine 0.5–1 mg. Neostigmine does not cross the blood–brain barrier.

52. a) True.
   b) True.
   c) False.   5 s.
   d) True.
   e) True.

53. a) True.
b) True.
c) False.
d) True.
e) True.
New England Journal of Medicine (1986) **315**: 1495–1500.

54. a) True.
b) True.
c) True.
d) True.
e) False.

55. a) False.
b) True.
c) False.
d) False.
e) False.

56. a) True.
b) False.
c) False.
d) False.
e) False.

57. a) False.
b) False.
c) True.
d) False.
e) False.

58. a) False.
b) False.
c) False.
d) True.
e) False.

59. a) True.
   b) False.
   c) False.
   d) False.
   e) False.

60. a) False.
   b) True.
   c) False.
   d) False.
   e) False.

OSCEs Questions

1. Comment on this set of results from a 40-year-old man admitted with abdominal pain and vomiting. What is the likely cause of these abnormalities?

   Na   128 mmol/l.
   K   3.1 mmol/l.
   Cl   85 mmol/l.
   HCO_3 36 mmol/l.
   Urea   7.2 mmol/l.
   Creatinine 90 µmol/l.

2. Comment on the following set of pulmonary function tests performed by a 30-year-old woman (height 145 cm) prior to anaesthesia.

	Baseline	*After inhaled salbutamol*
FEV_1	1.8 l	2.4 l
FVC	3.0 l	3.0 l
FEV_1/FVC	60%	80%
PEFR	220 l/min	350 l/min

3. The following results are from the full blood count of a 67-year-old woman who presented with weight loss and a pelvic mass.

   Hb   10.8 g/dl
   WBC 9.8×10^9 mm^3
   Pl 272×10^9 mm^3
   MCV   74 fl/dl
   MCHC   27 g/dl
   MCH   25 pg

   What abnormalities are present? What are the possible causes of this picture?

4. Comment on this set of arterial blood gas results.

H⁺   56 nmol/l (pH 7.25).
pCO₂   3.4 kPa.
pO₂   11.1 kPa.
BE   −13 mmol/l.
HCO₃stand   15 mmol/l.

5. Comment on this set of arterial blood gas results.

H⁺   73 nmol/1 (pH 7.18).
pCO₂   10.6 kPa.
pO₂   5.7 kPa.
HCO₃stand   26 mmol/l.
BE   −2 mmol/l.

6. What is shown in Figure 1? When should it be used? How should it be connected?

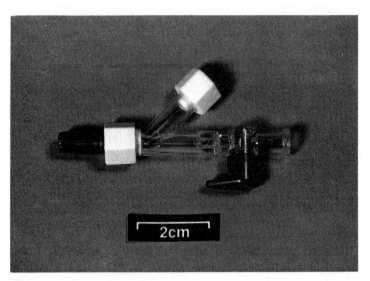

Figure 1

7. What is shown in Figure 2? In what group of patients is this indicated? How much air is required to inflate the cuff?

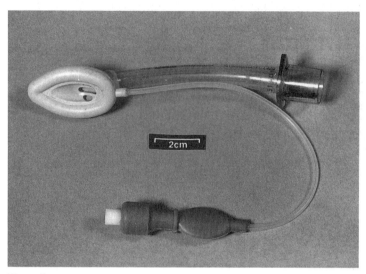

Figure 2

8. What is shown in Figure 3? What are its advantages?

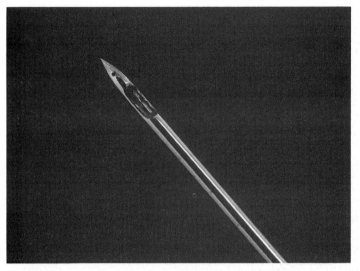

Figure 3

9. List the anatomical and physiological changes of relevance to anaesthesia which occur in pregnancy.

OSCEs Answers

1. Abnormalities:

Hyponatraemia.
Hypokalaemia.
Hypochloraemia.
Alkalosis.

There is a hypokalaemic, hypochloraemic metabolic alkalosis consistent with prolonged vomiting as a result of pyloric obstruction.

2. Abnormalities:

Reduced FEV_1.
Reduced FVC.
Reduced FEV_1/FVC ratio.
Reduced PEFR.

These results show an obstructive pattern which is largely reversible after inhaled bronchodilator and suggests asthma.

3. Abnormalities:

Anaemia.
Microcytosis.
Hypochromia – reduced MCHC.

This is the characteristic picture of iron deficiency anaemia.

Differential diagnosis:

Gastrointestinal blood loss from a neoplasm, ulcer or arteriovenous malformation.
Poor diet.
Small bowel disease, e.g. coeliac.

4. Abnormalities:

Acidosis.
Hypocarbia.
Low bicarbonate.
Large base deficit.

This is a metabolic acidosis with partial respiratory compensation from hyperventilation.

5. Abnormalities:

Acidosis.
Hypercarbia.
Hypoxia.

These results show an acute uncompensated respiratory acidosis.

6. This is a Cardiff anti-reflux valve. This or a similar device is required when intravenous fluids and an opioid infusion or patient-controlled analgesia are administered via the same intravenous cannula. In the event of the cannula becoming obstructed, the device will prevent reflux of opioid into the intravenous fluid with the potential risk of a subsequent uncontrolled bolus being administered to the patient. In this device the opioid infusion is connected to the side channel of the device and the intravenous fluids to the other.

7. This is a size 1 laryngeal mask airway. It is indicated in children of <1 year. The maximum volume of air required to inflate the cuff is 6 ml.

8. This is a 24G Sprotte needle. With its pencil point and side orifice it is one of a number of needles for lumbar puncture which are designed to split rather than cut dural fibres and reduce the incidence of post-dural puncture headache.

9. Mucosal oedema of the airway.

Reduced FRC, increased oxygen consumption, increased minute volume.

Increased circulating volume, increased heart rate, increased cardiac output, reduced blood pressure, reduced systemic vascular resistance, supine hypotensive syndrome.

Water and sodium retention, peripheral oedema.

Increased gastric acid production, incompetence of the oesophageal sphincter.

Reduced haematocrit, increased fibrinogen, tendency to thrombosis.

Index

N.B. Page references to questions and answers are prefixed by 'q' and 'a' respectively.

Abdominal pain and vomiting in 40-year-old man, abnormalities, q144, a148
Acetylcholine, q32, a46
Acetylsalicylic acid, see Aspirin
Addison's disease, q97, a111
Adenosine, q5, a20; q62, a77
ADH secretion, inappropriate, syndrome of, q39, a54
Adrenal cortex, q32, a46
Adrenal medulla, q60, a74
Airways, Mallampati classification, q93, a108
Alcohol, effects of chronic excess consumption, q94, a109
Aldosterone, q88, a102
Alfentanil, q5, a20
Altitude, acclimatization to 3500m of, q61, a75
Alveolar to arterial pO_2 gradient, q4, a19
Amethocaine, q7, a23
Aminoglycoside antibiotics, q4, a19
Anaphylaxis, q68, a83
Anion gap, q13, a28
Antidepressants, tricyclic, q37, a52
Aortic stenosis, q125, a141
Aprotinin, q34, a49
Arterial blood gas results, q145, a149
Arterial hypertension, q39, a54
Arterial to end-tidal pCO gradient, q115, a131
    where capnography in intubated patient, q116, a132
Arthritis, see Rheumatoid arthritis
Aspirin (acetylsalicylic acid)
    dose of 600–900 mg/day, q63, a79
    indications for, q6, a21
Atrial fibrillation, causes, q66, a81

Autonomic neuropathy, q9, a25
Axillary brachial plexus block, q93, a108

Bacterial endocarditis, q12, a28
Benzodiazepines, q6, a21; q36, a50
Bier's block, q39, a53
Bile acids, q61, a77
Blood gases, q11, a27; q145, a149
Blood pressure monitor, automatic oscillometric, q59, a74
Blood-brain barrier, drugs crossing, q36, a51; q119, a136
Bohr effect, q116, a132
Brachial plexus, q8, a24; q87, a101
Bronchial smooth muscle, q60, a75
Bronchiolitis, q96, a111
Bronchoconstriction, drugs causing, q90, a104
Bupivacaine
    cardiac arrest induced by, q97, a111
    caudal injection of, q120, a137
    toxicity, q123, a140

Calcitonin, q88, a102
Capnogram traces, q87, a101
Capnography, q59, a73; q88, a102
    in intubated patient, q88, a102; q116, 132
Captopril, q118, a135
Carcinoid tumours, q69, a84
Cardiac arrest
    features associated with good prognosis, q126, a142
    indications for sodium bicarbonate, q42, a57
    induced by bupivacaine, q97, a111

Cardiac cycle, q61, a76
Cardiac failure, congestive, q10, a26
Central anticholinergic syndrome, q125, a141
Cerebral perfusion pressure (CPP) after head injury q8, a23
Cerebrospinal fluid, normal, q89, a102
Charcoal, activated, q9, a25
Child
 1-year-old: characteristics, q32, a46
 3-year-old: nephrectomy, q6, a22; q65, a81
Cholestatic jaundice, drugs causing, q63, a79
Cimetidine, drug effects enhanced by chronic ingestion of, q91, a106
Circle system with vaporizer outside circle, using, q95, a110
Clonidine, q118, a134
CO₂ electrode, q68, a83
Coagulation factors, q3, q13; a18, a28
Cocaine intoxication, features, q125, a142
Combined oral contraceptive pill, results of taking, q122, a139
Conn's syndrome, q123, a140
Contraceptive pill, see Combined oral contraceptive pill
CPP (cerebral perfusion pressure) after head injury q8, a23
Cricoid pressure q94, a109
Cushing's syndrome, q67, a82
Cyclic AMP, q90, a104
 drugs acting by increasing intracellular, q90, a105
Cylinder supplies of anaesthetic gases, q121, a137
Cytochrome P450, q120, a136
 inhibitors, q36, a50

Day case anaesthesia and surgery, contraindications, q66, a82
Desflurane, q90, a105
Desmopressin acetate, q91, a105
Diabetes mellitus, q96, a111
Diabetes, non-insulin-dependent, q66, a82; q122, a139
Diabetes, non-insulin-dependent, and surgery, q10, a26
Diabetic ketoacidosis, q10, a25
Diazepam, q64, a80
Dopamine infusion at 4 µg/kg/h, q62, a77
Dopaminergic antagonists, q35, a50
Dopexamine, q119, a135

Down's syndrome, associations, q124, a141
Drug interactions
 likelihood of important, q91, a106
 resulting from pharmacokinetic factors, q35, a49
Duchenne muscular dystrophy, q98, a112
Dystrophica myotonica, q65, a80

ECG see Electrocardiogram
Ejection fraction, normal, q98, a112
Electrical potentials, biological, q58, a72
Electricity, q31, a45; q114, a130
 current at 50 Hz passing through body via skin contact, q69, a84
Electrocardiogram (ECG)
 12-lead, q2, a16; q59, a74
 Q waves on, q124, a141
Electroencephalography, q40, a55
 during anaesthesia, q124, a140
Electromyography, q99, a113
Elimination half life of drug, q35, a50
EMLA cream, q121, a137
Endobronchial intubation during anaesthesia, likely results of unnoticed, q120, a137
Endocarditis, bacterial, q12, a28
Endotracheal intubation
 features predictive of difficulty in, q121, a138
 minimizing pressor response to, q94, a109
Epidural injection, lumbar, q8, a23
Epidural opioids, respiratory depression after use of, q94, a109
Epiglottitis, q7, a22
Erythropoietin, q60, a75
Evoked potentials, measuring, q68, a84
Exponential function where t = time and K = the rate constant, q68, a84
Exponential processes, q86, a100

Fallot's tetralogy, features, q66, a82
Femoral nerve, q37, a52
Fentanyl, q5, a20
Fentanyl citrate, q34, a48; q62, a77
Fetal circulation, q116, a132
Fetal haemoglobin, q33, a47
First-order kinetics, q63, a78
5-Hydroxytryptamine, q34, a48; q90, a104

Fluids, flowing through tube of varying
    diameter, q1, a15
Flumazenil, q92, a107
F$_i$ O$_2$, devices supplying fixed, q95, a110
40% Ventimask, q31, a46
Fraction of false negatives, q128, a142
Fraction of false positives, q127, a142
Functional residual capacity, q117, a133

Gases
    characteristics, q58, a73
    critical temperatures, q86, a100
Gilbert's syndrome, q120, a136
Glass electrode, q70, a85
Glomerular filtration rate, q3, a17
Glomerular filtration rate,, substance used
    to measure, q60, a75
Glucose-6-phosphate dehydrogenase
    deficiency, q11, a26
Glucuronides, formation, q35, a49
Glutaraldehyde, 2%, q119, a136

Haemoglobin
    fetal, q33, a47
    S, q89, a103
Haemophilia A, q40, a55; q121, a138
Halothane, q36, a51; q65, a81
Head injury, cerebral perfusion pressure
    (CPP) after, q8, a23
Heparin, q5, a20
Hepatic blood flow
    decrease, q63, a79
    and drugs clearance, q64, a79; q92,
        a107
Humidity, q1, a15; q69, a84; q115, a131
Hypercalcaemia, causes, q67, a82
Hyperglycaemia, q92, a106
Hyperthermia, malignant, q37, a51
Hyperthyroidism, q67, a83
Hypokalaemia, q9, a24; q93, a108
Hypotension, vasodilatation and, drugs
    causing, q93, a108
Hypothermia, q70, a85
    cardiac effects, q13, a29
Hypothyroid patients, q123, a140
Hysterectomy, pulmonary embolism
    diagnosis after, q38, a53

Immunoglobulins, q61, a77; q117, a134
Insulin, q33, a48; q61, a76
    secretion stimulation q89, a104

Interleukin-6, systemic effects, q34, a48
Intra-tracheal administration route, drugs
    suitable for, q97, a111
Intrinsic and extrinsic pathways,
    coagulation factors, q3, a18
Iron deficiency anaemia, q38, a53
Isotopes of same element, q30, a44

Ketamine, q119, a135
Ketoacidosis, diabetic, q10, a25
Kidney, normal, q32, a47
Kinetics, first-order, q63, a78

Laminar flow, q114, a130
Laryngeal mask airway, q115, a131
    in children, q63, a79
Liquid manometers, q98, a112
Lumbar epidural injection, q8, a23
Lumbar puncture, q41, a55
Luteinizing hormone, q2, a17

Magnesium, q3, a18
Mallampati classification of airways, q93,
    a108
Manometers, liquid, q98, a112
Metabolic acidosis, and anion gap, q40,
    a55
Methaemoglobinaemia, q70, a85
    causes, q99, a112
Methionine synthetase, q95, a110
Methoxamine, q34, a48
Microcytic anaemia, causes, q64, a80
Milk, human, q115, a132
Morphine sulphate, q6, a21
    absorption routes, q94, a109
Multiple choice question examinations,
    sitting, ix
Muscular dystrophy, Duchenne, q98,
    a112
Myasthenia gravis, q123, a140
Myocardial infarction, q41, a56
Myocardial perfusion, q89, a103

Na$^+$/K$^+$-ATPase, q60, a74
Nasotracheal intubation q38, a52
Nausea and vomiting, postoperative, q8,
    24a
Negative predictive value, q129, a143
Neostigmine, q120, a136

Nephrectomy, 3-year-old, q6, a22; q65, a81
Nerve fibres, see Peripheral
Neurofibromatosis, associations, q41, a56
Neuropathy, autonomic, q9, a25
Neurotransmitters
    human, q2, a17; q4, a19
Neutrophils, characteristics, q4, a19
Newton, value, q12, a27
Nicotinic acetylcholine receptor, q116, a132
Nifedipine, q118, a134
Nitric oxide (NO), q38, a53; q65, a81; q125, a141
Nociceptive stimuli, transmission, q117, a133

1-deamino-8-D-arginine vasopressin, q91, a105
Oral contraceptive pill, see Combined oral contraceptive pill
Organophosphate insecticide poisoning, q42, a56
Osmosis, q58, a72
Oximeters, see Pulse oximetry
Oxygen, q30, a44
    delivery devices, q2, a16
Oxygen-haemoglobin dissociation curve, q3, a18

Pascal, q124, a140
Pathways, see Intrinsic and extrinsic pathways
PEEP (positive end expiratory pressure), application of 10 cm H_2O of, q92, a107
Peripheral nerve fibres, q117, a134
Peripheral nerve stimulator, q12, a27
Pharmacodynamic drug interactions, q5, a20
Phenothiazines, q37, a51
Phosphodiesterase inhibitors, q5, a20
Plasma cholinesterase, q69, a84
Platelet aggregation
    inhibition, q89, a103
    stimulation, q33, a47
Platelets, drugs impairing action of, q92, 107a
Pneumoperitoneum during laparoscopic cholecystectomy, q36, a51
pO_2 gradient, alveolar to arterial, q4, a19

Porphyria, q97, a112
    features of acute intermittent, q122, a139
Positive end expiratory pressure, see PEEP
Positive predictive value, q128, a143
Postoperative nausea and vomiting, q8, a24
Pre-eclampsia, requirements for diagnosis of, q122, a139
Pre-renal renal failure, q67, a83
Pregnancy
    blood in, q13, a28
    third trimester, q9, a25; q65, a81
Pregnancy, changes during, q147, a150
Prolactin, q2, a17
Prostate carcinoma, q39, a54
Pulmonary artery catheter, q59, a73
Pulmonary embolism diagnosis after hysterectomy, q38, a53
Pulmonary function tests, 30-year-old woman, q144, a148
Pulse oximetry, q1, a16; q11, a27
    spurious readings, q31, a45

Radioactivity, q86, a100
Regional anaesthesia, intravenous, q39, a53
Renal blood flow, q4, a18
Renal failure, features of chronic, q95, a110
Renal tubules, absorption, q3, a17
Respiratory depression after use of epidural opioids, q94, a109
Respiratory distress syndrome, adult (ARDS), features, q122, a138
Rheumatoid arthritis, q10, a26
    associations, q96, a110
Rheumatoid disease, q64, a80

Screening test for disease, q43, a57
Self-poisoning, treatment, 98, 112
Sensitivity, calculating, q127, a142
Serine proteases, q13, a28
Serotinin, q124, a141
Serum potassium concentration of 2.7 mmol/l, q38, a53
Sevoflurane, q118, a135
SI units, q40, a55
Sickle cell trait, q117, a133
Sleep, q87, a102
Soda lime, q118, a134

Sodium bicarbonate (8.4%), effects of intravenous, q13, a28
Solubility, q30, a44
Specificity, calculating, q126, a142
Sphygmomanometer, manual, q40, a54
Spinal canal, q7, a23
SpO_2 readings, inaccurate, q1, a16
Standard deviation, q70, a85
Statistical sensitivity, q71, a85
Statistical specificity of test, q99, a113
Statistics, q43, a57
Stomach, q87, a102
Stress response to surgery, q96, a111
Subarachnoid anaesthesia, q64, a80
   contraindications, q37, a52
Supine patients, q12, a27
Surface tension, q87, a101
Surgery, stress response to, q96, a111
Suxamethonium, q121, a137

Temperature, physical principles used to measure, q114, a131
Testosterone, q32, a46
Thalassaemia, q41, a56
Thoracic epidural analgesia, q42, a56
Thrombin, q33, a47

Thrombosis after surgery, deep venous, q7, a22
Transdermal absorption, drugs effective after, q93, a108
Tubular necrosis, acute, q11, a26
12-lead ECG, normal recording, q59, a74

Variance, q14, a29
Vasodilatation and hypotension, drugs causing, q93, a108
Vecuronium, q62, a78
Venous pressure waveform, central, q31, 45
Ventimask, 40%, q31, a46
Verapamil, q7, a23
Vital capacity, components, q33, a48
Vitamin B_{12} deficiency, causes, q9, a24
Volatile anaesthetics, q6, a22
von Willebrand's disease, q67, a83
von Willebrand's factor, q42, a56

Warfarin, q91, a105
   patient taking, q62, a78
Weight loss and a pelvic mass, 67-year-old woman, q144, a148